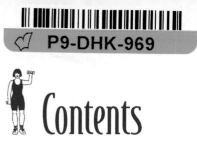

Contents

Acknowledgments

We gratefully acknowledge the contributions of William D. McArdle, Ph.D., Queens College, New York; Karen Miller-Kovach, M.S., R.D., Weight Watchers International; Bud Rockhill, for Cardio-Fitness Corporations, New York; John Wildman and Andrew Smith, The Fitness Institute, Toronto.

Foreword

I applaud Weight Watchers International for the publication of its new *Complete Exercise Book*.

By any criteria, obesity is a major health problem. Unfortunately, we are in the midst of an epidemic of obesity in the United States. During the period between 1980 and 1991, the number of obese adults in America grew by a shocking 31 percent. One out of three adults in our society is now at least 20 percent above his or her desirable weight.

A sedentary lifestyle is a major cause of obesity in the United States. For many Americans, physical inactivity may be a more significant factor in the development and maintenance of excess body weight than is the consumption of extra calories. A planned program of increased physical activity, therefore, is a critical component of any weight-management program.

Not only is physical activity a key component of healthy weight management, it also yields many other significant health benefits. Individuals who participate in consistent physical activity throughout their lives significantly lower their risk of heart disease, certain forms of cancer, diabetes, and hypertension. In addition, they slow the process of osteoporosis, reduce stress, and improve their mood. Exercise is good medicine!

We are entering an era in which individuals are recognizing that weight management is a *health* issue. As a physician, I have always admired Weight Watchers common sense, scientifically based approach to healthy weight loss, and lifelong weight management. *The Weight Watchers Complete Exercise Book* follows the same motivational, practical approach for which the organization has become famous. This is a fine book and one that will help its readers become more active, control their weight, and lead healthier lives!

James M. Rippe, M.D.

WEIGHT WATCHERS

Since 1963, Weight Watchers has grown from a handful of people to millions of enrollments annually. Today, Weight Watchers is the recognized leading name in safe and sensible weight control. Weight Watchers members are a diverse group from youths, 10 years old and over, to senior citizens, attending meetings virtually around the globe.

Growing numbers of people purchase and enjoy our popular, expanding line of convenience foods, best-selling cookbooks, personal calendar planners and audio and video tapes. Weight loss and weight management results vary by individual, but we recommend that you attend Weight Watchers meetings, follow the Weight Watchers Food Plan, and participate in regular physical activity. Consult your physician before following the advice or performing the exercises/activities presented here. For the Weight Watchers meeting nearest you, call 1-800-651-6000.

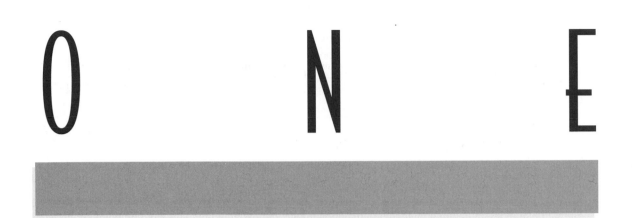

How You'll Benefit from Exercise

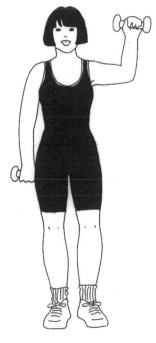

Physical fitness has become a priority for people of all ages—and for good reason! Until recently, many people began a fitness program only to achieve a beautiful body or a perfect "10." That's too daunting for most people, however, and it isn't even the real role of exercise. Improvements in your health and your ability to complete everyday tasks, to function effectively in stressful and demanding situations, and improved appearance are the real advantages of regular exercise. People who exercise regularly will tell you they enjoy it—even look forward to it! The benefits they reap range from improved health to a leaner, trimmer look, to an improved quality of life.

Improved Health

Some people have the mistaken belief that for exercise to be beneficial, they must endure long, hard, daily exercise sessions, as if training to run a marathon. However, recent research has revealed that going to this extreme level of training is not necessary to improve overall health. Actually, over the past few years it's been discovered that even relatively modest levels of physical activity can make a great impact on your health.

In fact, in the early 1990s the American Heart Association upgraded physical inactivity from its list of contributing factors for cardiovascular disease to the more powerful category of primary risk factor. Physical inactivity joined smoking, high blood pressure, and elevated blood cholesterol as one of the strongest predictors of cardiovascular disease.

In 1993 a group of experts from the U.S. Centers for Disease Control and Prevention and the American College of Sports Medicine announced that regular, moderate-intensity physical activity results in substantial health benefits. In fact, the experts issued the following recommendation:

> *Every American adult should accumulate 30 minutes or more of moderate-intensity physical activity over the course of most days of the week.*

You'll find that regular exercise has many merits:

◆ Reducing your risk of developing heart disease, adult-onset diabetes, hypertension, and certain cancers
◆ Favorably modifying your blood lipid (cholesterol) profile
◆ Slowing the loss of bone mass (osteoporosis) associated with aging
◆ Burning calories and aiding your efforts to lose or control body weight without having to rely solely on limiting caloric intake
◆ Conserving muscle (lean tissue) if you're attempting to lose weight
◆ Promoting mental well-being—reducing anxiety, mild to moderate

depression, tension, and stress. In addition, exercise has a positive effect on self-esteem.

It's easy to see why it makes sense to exercise. You get a lot back from developing regular exercise habits. And the good news for all of us is that our bodies respond quite favorably to exercise at any age!

The First Goal—Don't Be Sedentary

An important point about exercise: You don't have to join a gym, sweat buckets, or run miles in order to gain from a workout.

Your goal is to be sure your lifestyle isn't sedentary. In fact, when it comes to health, the greatest benefits to be found are for those individuals who were previously sedentary, who make the transition to become moderate exercisers. You don't have to be an athlete to reap the major benefits of physical activity!

Do you lead a sedentary lifestyle? If some of the following statements accurately describe your habits, consider yourself sedentary.

◆ Recreational activities such as walking, swimming, cycling, or dancing are rare occurrences.

◆ The majority of your leisure time is spent in sedentary or low-energy level activities such as watching TV or movies, reading, or visiting with friends.

◆ You have a real desk job. During most of the time you are at work, you're seated at your desk or in meetings.

◆ Work around the house (typical household chores, yardwork, etc.) is infrequent and not particularly labor intensive. Your spouse, children, or hired help do the "real" chores.

◆ To move from one point to another you generally rely on your car instead of walking, on an elevator rather than stairs.

Sound familiar? If so, don't worry. Adding regular exercise to your life really can be easy!

All Exercise Is Not Alike

While many forms of exercise provide similar benefits, no one exercise or activity does everything. Some exercises are best suited to improving the strength and tone of muscles, others enhance the flexibility of muscles and joints, still others condition the cardiovascular system while burning a significant number of calories. Which form of exercise is most appropriate for you? To help you answer this question, read the following description of each component of physical fitness and how it can be improved.

The Components of Fitness

What Is Flexibility?

Flexibility is the ability to move the joints of your body through their full range of motion without stress, injury, or pain. It means that your muscles, tendons, and joints are supple and loose. Muscles that are supple are less likely to be pulled or injured.

How Can You Improve Your Flexibility?

You can improve your flexibility by doing proper stretching exercises.

What Is Aerobic Fitness?

Aerobic or cardiovascular fitness enables you to perform vigorous, continuous activity (such as walking, jogging, swimming, or biking) without undue fatigue and to recover rapidly when you've stopped exercising. Aerobic fitness is highly dependent on the capacity of your lungs, heart, and blood vessels to deliver oxygen to exercising muscles.

How Do You Improve Your Aerobic Fitness?

You improve by exercising large muscle groups in a continuous and rhythmic manner (as in walking, swimming, or dancing). The exercise need not be strenuous, but it should be performed at moderate intensity for at least 20 to 30 minutes per session.

What Is Muscular Strength?

Muscular strength is your muscles' ability to exert themselves against resistance—whether that resistance comes from weights, water (as in swimming), or even carrying groceries! Strong, toned muscles maintain proper posture and also add an attractive shape to the body.

How Do You Improve Muscular Strength?

Strength or resistance training is based on the principle that your muscles become stronger when you challenge them to work harder. Physiologists call this level of training "overload." Strength-training or resistance-training exercises are designed to isolate specific muscles in the body. For example, curl-ups isolate, and therefore tone and strengthen, the abdominal muscles.

What Is Calorie-Burning Exercise?

While all exercise burns calories, calorie-burning workouts are designed to maximize this effect. They rely on the continuous rhythmic contraction of the large muscles of your arms or legs (or both together). The intensity is kept light to moderate, which allows for extended workouts and significant calorie burning.

How Can You Burn More Calories?

You can burn more calories by increasing your participation in activities that involve the continuous rhythmic movement of large muscle groups. Walking and dancing are both excellent calorie-burning exercises.

What Are Your Fitness Goals?

As you've just read, all exercise is not alike. Each component of fitness is different and each contributes in a unique way to your body's overall health and well-being.

How can you learn what kind of exercise is best suited to your needs? Take the short self-assessment quiz below; it's designed to help you identify your fitness goals.

Read each statement. If it describes your present condition, check the *Agree* box. If the statement does not describe your present condition, check the *Disagree* box. To determine the workout that's best for you, use the following guidelines:

◆ If you check two or more Agree boxes in any one category—do the workout for that category.

◆ If you check two or more Agree boxes in more than one category—do the Overall Fitness Workout (page 99).

Aerobic Workout (page 81)

	Agree	Disagree
◆ Even a moderate bout of physical activity (for example, climbing several flights of stairs or walking continuously for 5 to 10 minutes) leaves me winded or short of breath.	❏	❏
◆ Aerobic activities such as walking, cycling, or dancing cause my heart to race and leave me winded.	❏	❏
◆ Yardwork or household chores often leave me feeling winded and fatigued.	❏	❏
◆ Recreational activities such as hiking, swimming, or dancing leave me fatigued and limit my ability to enjoy these activities.	❏	❏

Flexibility and Relaxation Workout (page 67)

◆ My muscles and joints often feel tight or stiff.	❏	❏
◆ My doctor has told me that my low back problems are attributable to being "out of shape"—*not* the result of an injury or a congenital abnormality.	❏	❏
◆ I have a high degree of stress in my life with multiple demands on my time from family, work, and social responsibilities.	❏	❏
◆ Tight muscles or stiff joints make participation in recreational activities or household chores uncomfortable or painful.	❏	❏

Calorie-Burning Workout (page 39)

◆ I don't really eat that much, but I still find it difficult to keep from gaining weight.	❏	❏
◆ My present weight is 10 or more pounds above a weight I would feel comfortable with.	❏	❏
◆ Even when I follow a reduced-calorie food plan, I find it difficult to keep from gaining weight.	❏	❏

◆ I know I have to follow a reduced-calorie food
plan to lose weight, but I would also like to improve my fitness.   ❏   ❏

Toning and Strengthening Workout (page 51)

◆ I am presently at or near a personal goal weight
and desire more shapely, toned muscles.   ❏   ❏

◆ I lack the muscular strength to enjoy participating
in and improving my skills in recreational activities
(for example, tennis or skiing).   ❏   ❏

◆ I would like to gain a bit more strength in the
muscles throughout my body.   ❏   ❏

◆ I find that as I lose weight, my muscles seem to feel
soft and out of shape.   ❏   ❏

T W O

Staying Motivated

How to Stick with an Exercise Program

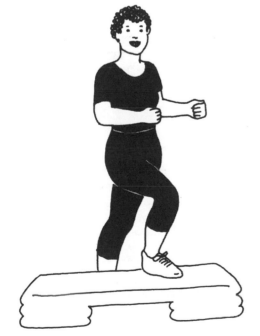

People often start an exercise program with great enthusiasm, then lose steam. However, you *can* keep your motivation high and continue your exercise program with the support you'll find here.

The first thing to realize about motivation and exercise is that *everyone* needs it. It's the rare individual who doesn't need a push to exercise at one time or another. Knowing that you're not alone in needing encouragement can help you get going when you feel unmotivated.

Four-Step Action Plan to Get Moving

Let's get moving! It's important to set realistic goals and create a specific plan of attack. Beginners often set their goals too high; they don't realize that getting fit takes time and effort. In fact, it's easier to adopt an active lifestyle in small increments than to make drastic changes so different from your usual routine that they can't be maintained for long.

These four steps will help you enjoy a more active lifestyle:

Step 1. Determine Your Current Level of Physical Activity

How active are you every day? During the course of a typical week? To focus your attention on specific habits and opportunities, review the chart in Chapter 11, page 134.

Step 2. Once You Have a Feel for Your Current Level of Activity, Set a Simple, Short-Term Goal for Yourself

When setting this goal, don't think in terms of "everyday," "from now on," or "all the time." Often, these kinds of words (or "absolutes") signify that your goal is too challenging. Similarly, don't set your goal too far into the future. A good time frame for a short-term goal is this week. As an extra incentive, record your original activity level and your weekly goals in the Personal Fitness Planner (pages 132–33) at the back of this book.

Looking for suggestions about setting short-term goals? Try out the following ideas.

If your daily routine is fairly sedentary, and doesn't include exercise or much physical activity, try one of the following as an initial goal:

◆ Walk for 15 minutes during your lunch break at least three times a week.

◆ Do one of the workouts in this book at least two times this week.

◆ Participate in some form of physical activity—walking, cycling, hiking, yardwork—with friends or family for one day during the weekend.

◆ Register for an introductory class in an activity you might enjoy (swimming, dance classes, jogging, self-defense, etc.).

If your weekly routine already includes some form of physical activity, try to do more. Here are some realistic goals for any given week:

◆ Boost your total weekly mileage by walking three miles more than you did last week.

◆ Add 15 minutes to your usual workout (try one of the workouts in this book, go biking or swimming, etc.).

◆ Try to do your typical workout in less time. For example, if walking your usual route takes 30 minutes, walk a little faster (at a higher intensity) and complete the walk in less than 30 minutes.

Step 3. Figure Out What You Need to Do to Accomplish Your Goal

This important step is often omitted, although it holds the key to increasing the likelihood you'll exercise. This step involves asking yourself what you can do beforehand to increase the chances that you'll exercise later.

Want to take an aerobics class? First find out where and when classes are taught and choose one that best fits your schedule. Planning a walk during your lunch hour? Make sure you bring comfortable walking shoes to work. Taking a bike ride this weekend? Make sure your bike is tuned up; it's not pleasant to ride an uncomfortable or unsafe bicycle.

Planning ahead is easy to do, especially when you see how much it increases the likelihood you'll exercise. Get to know what you need to do beforehand to make exercise part of your weekly routine.

Step 4. Reward Yourself When You Reach a Goal

At the end of the week, examine your results. When you reach a goal, congratulate yourself! An appropriate reward for a real milestone or a long-term goal may be a gift to yourself, such as a new pair of sneakers, a massage, or a new workout outfit. Any kind of small nonfood reward will be a pleasant treat. Meanwhile, you may find that the best reward for short-term goals is the feeling of making positive changes in your life. Enjoy how good it feels to exercise, and how proud you feel when you accomplish what you set out to do.

Going Forward—A Progression Strategy

As your fitness improves, you'll want to set new, more challenging goals. When you're comfortable with your new activity level, it's time to take another look at your daily routine. Can you fit in more activity? Can you build on to the level of activity you've already reached? Remember that drastic changes to your physical activity cannot be maintained as easily as small, modest challenges. If you become so excited by your progress that you jump ahead dramatically in duration, frequency, or intensity of a workout, you could become discouraged or even injure yourself and then lose ground by missing workouts.

When one of the following statements describes your current exercise program, you'll know it's time to set a new, more challenging goal:

◆ This is getting too easy.

◆ I believe I can comfortably handle more.

◆ My schedule permits me to set aside more time for physical activity.

Setting a more challenging goal may involve one of the following:

◆ Beginning a new type of workout

◆ Increasing the length of your workout

◆ Doing the workout more frequently

◆ Increasing the intensity of the workout

Increase Your Ability to Succeed

How many times have you decided to begin exercising on a regular basis? You start out full of energy and enthusiasm, but find after a few weeks you're back where you started—not exercising regularly. Experts cite two reasons for this common occurrence—a lack of social support and the absence of tangible results. To increase your ability to succeed, take these two important steps:

1. Seek the Support of Others

Throughout the day, a variety of different responsibilities (work, home, social, and personal) compete for your time and attention. Without the support of others, making time in your schedule for exercise can cause conflicts. Here are some suggestions for bolstering your social support at home and at the gym:

◆ Seek the support of individuals who have expressed concern for your health and well-being in the past. Explain your goal and let them know your strategy for reaching it. For example, if you would like to go for a walk after dinner, explain that you would appreciate a hand with the cleanup.

◆ Recruit an exercise partner. Make plans to exercise with family or friends. Take advantage of the fact that many of us are more likely to honor a commitment made to others rather than one made to our-selves.

◆ Tap into the motivational support of an exercise group. Just as you may have developed a "sense of belonging" to other groups in the past, you might enjoy the camaraderie of a walking group, dance class, or other group exercise activity.

2. Focus on the Immediate Benefits of Exercise

While your primary motivation to exercise may be fueled by a desire to look good, feel good, or improve your health, you can't rush mother nature. The biological changes that result from regular exercise habits—stronger, more shapely muscles, reduced body fat, and an improved cardiovascular risk pro-file, among others—take time. While some changes happen sooner than oth-ers, weeks are the appropriate time frame in which to measure your progress, not days.

Meanwhile, it's easy to question the benefits of exercise as you work hard to make time in your schedule and are not rewarded by the results you seek. Rec-ognize this fact: you won't see the results you desire overnight. During the early days and weeks of your program, before any of the long-term training effects are apparent, focus your attention on the immediate, easily attainable benefits exercise can provide.

◆ Focus on how good it feels to take charge and make positive lifestyle changes. Taking the time to schedule exercise into your life is a challenge. It can require changing old habits, setting new priorities, and taking charge. Making positive life changes will make you feel empowered and rewarded! It will bolster your self-confidence in all areas of your life!

◆ Give yourself another reason to look forward to exercise. If the follow-ing ideas don't motivate you, use them to spark other ideas that may be more appropriate to your situation:

Capitalize on the social aspects of working out with others. Whether you invite a friend to join you for a walk or make new friends in a dance class, you'll have another reason for looking forward to getting out and exercising.

Appreciate the "escape" exercise provides. While exercising with others can be rewarding, most of us also appreciate time to be alone. Exercising by yourself can provide you with a block of time to collect your thoughts, figure out solutions to everyday prob-lems, or rejuvenate yourself by daydreaming.

Exercise Is Mind-Set

You've decided to commit yourself to an exercise program. How can you help yourself stay determined to exercise? Use these suggestions.

Make an Appointment with Yourself

You make doctor's appointments and set dates to see family and friends. Why not try thinking of your workout as an appointment with yourself? Note the date and time of your workout on your calendar. Just as you would with any other appointment, don't let other things get in the way. When you become as serious about keeping your workout "appointments" as everything else in your life, you know you're really committed.

See Exercise As Your Time

Some people fall into a trap of feeling guilty about working out. They feel as though exercise takes them away from family and friends and the millions of things they should be doing. Instead, try to think of exercise as your time—as time especially set aside to promote your health, time you deserve. Remember, too, that working out revitalizes you and will give you renewed energy and attention for work, friends, and family.

Use a Positive Mind-Set to Get Yourself Through the Workout

If during the whole time you're exercising you're thinking about when you'll be through, or thinking negative thoughts such as "I can't do this," or "I should be doing something more productive," you won't be helping yourself. Instead, think positive thoughts: how great you'll feel after the workout, how relaxed, self-confident, and invigorated. Remind yourself that these very qualities improve your ability to perform effectively in everyday situations that are stressful and demanding.

Choose Activities You Enjoy

Select the activity that gives you the most enjoyment. Don't feel compelled to choose an activity simply because it's popular or because other people you know happen to enjoy it. It's important to choose an activity that pleases you. If you don't like what you're doing, chances are you won't stick with it.

Don't Be Too Hard on Yourself

If your initial attempts at becoming more active are not working out, examine your experience. How can you improve your chances of succeeding? For example, if getting up a half hour earlier for a walk is not a viable option for you, then concentrate your exercise efforts during other times of the day. There is no one best approach to developing regular exercise habits and no one best time to exercise. Find what works for you. Put what doesn't work behind you and set your sights on new exercise goals.

Don't Compare Yourself to Others

The only true measure of your progress is comparing your activity level now to what it was before starting your exercise program. Don't fall into the trap of comparing yourself to anyone else. The activities they do, and the frequency, intensity, and duration of their exercise sessions, are not relevant to your success.

Beat Boredom

If you find exercise boring, you're unlikely to do it on a regular basis. Do what's necessary to make it more stimulating. Consider the following boredom-beating tips:

- ◆ Listen to a personal audio-cassette player or radio while exercising.
- ◆ Watch television while using a piece of home exercise equipment.
- ◆ Vary your activity. Bicycle during one workout, walk on the treadmill during the next. Do as many activities as you enjoy and make sense for your schedule.
- ◆ Learn a new skill. Take a tennis, swimming, or ski lesson.
- ◆ Sign up for a dance or a toning class.
- ◆ Join a gym or health club.
- ◆ Recruit an exercise partner or personal trainer.
- ◆ Buy a book stand for your stationary bicycle.
- ◆ Join a mall walking group.

Keeping Records and Measuring Success

You may find that it helps to keep a record of the progress you make in your exercise program. That way you can keep track of where you started, the goals you set, and how you achieved them. See Chapter 11, which contains a Personal Fitness Planner for you to keep a written record of your progress.

Keeping a written record of your exercise program is an excellent way of tracking your progress and giving you a tangible measure of your achievements.

The Positive Experience of Achieving Goals Will Spread into Everything You Do

Setting goals and reaching them will have a positive impact on you. You'll feel increased confidence and self-esteem because of what you've been able to do. These positive feelings will spread over into other areas of your life. You may find that you're not as likely to say "I can't do that" when it comes to trying out other sports, recreational activities, or more challenging projects at work.

Instead, you'll remind yourself that if you can exercise on a regular basis, or attain any other of your fitness goals, you can do anything else you set your mind to.

T H R E E

Getting Off on the Right Foot

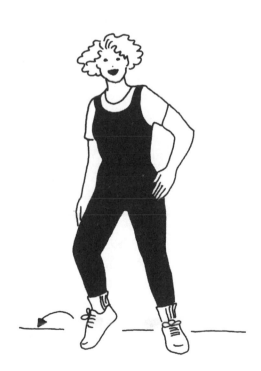

Before starting your exercise program, there are a few basics you'll want to know. What should the workout feel like? How will you know how hard to work? What should you wear? What kind of athletic shoes will you need? The answers to these questions will help you get your exercise program off to a good start.

How Hard Do You Need to Exercise? Learning to Pace Yourself

How do you know how much effort to put into exercise? How do you know how hard to work? First, you'll need to learn how to exercise at a pace that's comfortable, safe, and effective for you. The first guideline to follow relies strongly on common sense: Always listen to your body. It's usually quite good at letting you know if you're working too hard, or not hard enough.

The Talk Test

When participating in activities that are aerobic in nature such as dancing, walking, jogging, or cycling, the "talk test" is an easy way to determine if you're exercising at an appropriate level. Can you carry on a normal conversation during the workout? You should be able to. If you're breathing so hard that you can't speak normally, it means you're working too hard and should slow down. Expect your breathing to be increased during a workout, but you should be breathing comfortably at all times.

The Rate Your Activity Chart

The Rate Your Activity Chart is another helpful way of determining how hard you're working. It also enables you to determine if you're working at an appropriate level. Using the chart will help you determine how strenuous the exercise feels.

Take a look at the chart. While exercising, rate how hard the exercise is. This feeling should reflect your total amount of exertion, combining all sensations of physical stress, effort, and fatigue. Try not to concern yourself with any one factor. Instead, concentrate on your *total* feeling of exertion. Use the distinctions provided by the chart to determine your rating.

- ◆ Very Light
- ◆ Fairly Light
- ◆ Somewhat Hard
- ◆ Hard
- ◆ Very Hard

When you're just beginning a workout (during the warm-up), you should aim for "Very Light" or "Fairly Light"—anything higher indicates you're working too hard. Once you are in the main body of the workout, you should strive to

What Exercise Should Feel Like

It's important to have an idea of what exercise should feel like, so you know what to expect during and after a workout. With these general guidelines in mind, you'll have more control over your workout and your exercise program.

During and After Exercise
It's Okay to Feel:

◆ An increased heart rate (pulse) during exercise, which gradually returns to normal afterward

◆ A mild stretching or pulling feeling in the working muscles and joints while exercising

◆ An increased, but comfortable, rate of breathing during exercise, which gradually returns to normal when the session is over

◆ Mild perspiration

◆ Mild muscle soreness a day or two after exercising

◆ Mild fatigue after exercising, but if you must rest you've pushed too hard

It's Not Okay to Feel:

◆ Irregular heartbeat (pulse), particularly if your heartbeat was regular before you began exercising*

◆ Pain or pressure in your chest, neck, jaw, or arms*

◆ Unusual or extreme shortness of breath*

◆ Nausea, dizziness, cold sweating, or fainting*

◆ Chronic joint or muscle pain* *

* If you experience any of these symptoms, stop exercising and sit or lie down. Contact your physician promptly.

* * If persistent, contact your physician.

work at a level you would rate as "Somewhat Hard." If the activity feels harder than that, with a rating of "Hard" or "Very Hard," you're pushing too much. As you approach the end of the workout (during the cool-down), you should once again be able to rate the exercise as "Very Light" or "Fairly Light."

One helpful way to remember these distinctions: Always aim for middle ground during the main body of a workout, and begin and end each workout with much less effort.

Once you've learned to listen to your body, you'll automatically be able to find these points of distinction; for example, you'll know what "Somewhat Hard" feels like without thinking about it. Remember, if you ever feel pain or discomfort during a workout, slow down. If the pain persists, stop the activity immediately.

Clothing Corner—Indoor Workout Wear

What are the most important guidelines for choosing workout clothes? They should be lightweight and loose-fitting. If your clothing is too tight, or the fabric is too heavy, it will hamper your movements, and may cause overheating. Always make sure your exercise clothing fits appropriately and is comfortable.

Favor any lightweight and loose-fitting clothing that permits your skin to breathe. This allows perspiration to evaporate, which helps cool your body. Any clothing that retards the evaporation of perspiration (for example, heavy sweat suits or rubber/plastic suits) can cause dangerous overheating and should not be worn!

If you're not comfortable in a leotard or other trendy exercise clothing, don't wear them. A pair of shorts and a T-shirt are just fine.

As your fitness level improves, you may find that you become more interested in workout clothes that are designed for comfort and flexibility while you move. You may find that you want to try biking shorts or a leotard. If at first you don't feel comfortable in a leotard, try wearing a big T-shirt over it. As exercise becomes a part of your life, reward yourself with fashionable workout clothes.

Selecting an Exercise Shoe

While lightweight and loose-fitting are the main criteria for choosing exercise clothing, there is more to consider in selecting the right exercise shoe. An improper fit, or the wrong kind of shoe, can cause injury.

Use these guidelines for determining proper fit:

- From the moment you put them on, athletic shoes should be comfortable.
- Watch out that the shoes aren't too tight. Your feet will expand when you exercise, especially when you work out in hot weather.
- When trying on athletic shoes, wear the kind of socks you'll be wearing when you exercise.
- Make sure the inside surfaces of the shoes are free of exposed seams. These can irritate your feet or cause blisters.
- The sole of the shoe should flex easily where your foot bends, that is, at the ball of the foot.
- The shoes should support the arches of your feet.
- You should be able to wiggle your toes freely.
- There should be a space (about a finger's width) between the tip of your longest toe and the inside of each shoe.
- Your heels should fit snugly in the shoes.
- The collar of the shoe should not press uncomfortably against your ankle.
- Try on both shoes and walk around the store in them before you purchase a pair.

Which Shoe for Which Workout or Sport?

These days exercise shoes are designed with specific activities in mind. It is good to have an idea about the specifics of these activities so you can make a wise decision when selecting a shoe.

For Step Aerobics and Aerobic Dance Workouts

Because these activities often involve dance steps, aerobic dance shoes are lightweight and designed to provide extra support for side-to-side movements. Aerobic dance places stress on the front of the foot, so be sure to evaluate the shock-absorbing ability (cushioning) at this part of the shoe.

For Walking or Jogging

If you're planning to walk on a regular basis or for extended periods of time, it's important to invest in a good pair of walking shoes. Walking shoes are lightweight with breathable uppers and cushioning that gradually thickens at the heel to about twice the thickness of the front of the shoe. Tall or heavy people should look for shoes with the greatest amount of cushioning. Ask the salesperson to show you a variety of shoes so you can assess the difference in cushioning.

Even though jogging and walking shoes possess similar characteristics, if and when you decide to jog, invest in a pair of quality running shoes. Not only will they decrease the chances of discomfort or injury, but they will make jogging more pleasurable. Jogging is more stressful on your joints than walking and requires a shoe capable of withstanding the additional demands. Look for all the features of a walking shoe (see above) as well as extra cushioning and overall sturdier construction.

For Toning and Strengthening Workouts

Since toning and strengthening exercises are done in a stationary position, any kind of comfortable athletic shoe with support is appropriate.

More Than One Workout?

If you plan to participate in a variety of activities, consider purchasing a pair of "cross-trainers." These shoes combine characteristics of many types of shoes and are suitable for use in a variety of activities.

Preparing for a Home Workout

Before you begin exercising, you'll need to find appropriate space in your home. Look for an uncluttered area of your living room, bedroom, or den where you'll have a clear space and won't be hampered by furniture. You can move a lightweight table or chair out of the way to give yourself enough space. You'll probably want to choose a room where you can be alone, or a time of day when you won't be disturbed by other family members.

The basement can be a good spot if you're planning to do the Toning and Strengthening Workout. Any of the other workouts that include dance steps should not be done on the concrete floors found in most basements, since dancing on a concrete floor puts too much stress on your bones and joints. Exercising on carpet is fine, as long as it's not movable (stay off throw rugs) and the thickness is not so great as to cause you to trip (stay off shag rugs). Regardless of the flooring, always wear your athletic shoes.

Access to a stereo or CD player is also a plus, so you'll be able to listen to music while you work out.

Selecting Music

This is a chance to add a personal touch to your workout—music can make it fun to exercise. You can catch the beat and let your body move in time to the music. Not only does this feel good, but it also helps to get you into the rhythm of the moves. The beat of the music will determine how slow or fast you move and, in part, determine the intensity of your workout. For example, if you're working out to music that's 120 to 130 beats per minute, you'll move more slowly than you would working out to music that's 150 beats per minute. Step workouts are usually done to a catchy tune that has about 120 beats per minute; often the music used during step aerobics is slower than music used during aerobic dance.

Start out by checking your favorite dance tunes and see if they're right for the workout. Movie or theater soundtracks are often full of good choices—such as *The Big Chill* or *Stand by Me*. You can purchase tapes, such as those by Motown artists, that could have a series of appropriate sequential workout music. Either make your own tape, or use one you already own.

You'll need songs with a slower beat for the warm-up and cool-down. Try a song like "(I've Had) The Time of My Life," which is the love theme from *Dirty Dancing*. This song has under 120 beats per minute. "I Heard It Through the Grapevine" or "Yesterday" are also under 120 beats per minute. Songs with a fast beat are more appropriate for the body of the workout: for example, "Come See About Me" (about 125 beats per minute) or even songs with a faster beat like "Material Girl" (about 140 beats per minute) or "Papa's Got A Brand New Bag" (about 136 beats per minute). Popular songs like "Billy Jean" or "Like a Virgin" (about 120 beats per minute) are good for step workouts.

Use the following guidelines when choosing appropriate music for your workout:

WORKOUT TYPE OR SEGMENT	MUSIC SPEED (beats per minute)
Stretching	100 or less
Cardiovascular Warm-up and Cool-down	100 to 120
Step Aerobics	118 to 126
Aerobic Dance	120 to 150

Ready for Exercise?

Before you get started with any exercise program, you should have a checkup with your physician to make sure you are in good health. It's also important to discuss any exercise restrictions your doctor may have for you. To help you get a general idea as to whether you're ready to exercise, take a few minutes to answer these questions:

1. Has your physician ever said you have a heart problem or suspected a cardiac condition of any type?   Yes   No

2. Do you now have or have you ever had

    ◆ pressure, pain, or tightness in the chest brought on by exertion?   Yes   No

    ◆ bouts of irregular or uneven heart action?   Yes   No

    ◆ fainting spells or severe dizziness?   Yes   No

    ◆ diabetes or high blood pressure?   Yes   No

    ◆ high cholesterol, triglyceride, or high "lipids" or fats in your blood?   Yes   No

3. Has your blood pressure been high enough to require medication, now or in the past?   Yes   No

4. Has any close blood relative (parents, siblings, children) had a heart attack or stroke, under the age of 50?   Yes   No

5. Do you smoke more than $1^1/_2$ packs of cigarettes a day?   Yes   No

6. Are you a smoker (more than 15 cigarettes daily) who also takes birth-control pills?   Yes   No

7. Are you more than 50 pounds overweight?   Yes   No

8. Do you have any bone, joint, muscular, or vein problems (such as arthritis, rheumatism, gout, bad back, or very bad leg veins)?   Yes   No

9. Are you over 65 and not accustomed to vigorous exercise?   Yes   No

10. Are you pregnant?   Yes   No

11. Does walking up one flight of stairs make you short of breath?   Yes   No

12. Is there any physical reason not mentioned here that would prevent you from following an activity program?   Yes   No

If You Answered Yes to One or More Questions . . .

Consult your physician before getting started on this, or any other exercise plan.

If You Answered No to One or More Questions . . .

You can be reasonably sure that you are physically ready to begin an exercise program. Just the same, checking with your physician before increasing your physical activity is a good idea.

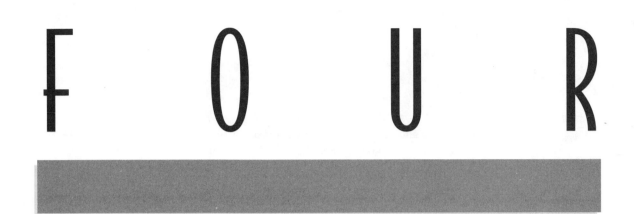

F O U R

Warm-ups and Cool-downs

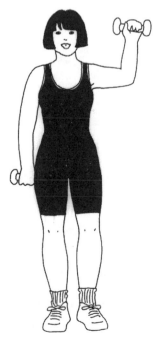

Warming up before you begin exercising, and cooling down after a workout, are important parts of every exercise session, so don't skip them! The warm-up and cool-down don't have to take long; about five to seven minutes is all the time they require. Understanding the purpose of the

27

warm-up and cool-down will help you perform them safely and effectively.

The Warm-up

It is recommended that every session of exercise—whether it's a stretching, strengthening and toning, or aerobic activity—begin with a warm-up. It's also suggested that you warm up before sports or recreational activities.

The goal of a warm-up is to get your body ready for the workout to come—it literally "warms up" the body. Warm-ups usually consist of two activities: some type of rhythmic movement that gets the heart pumping and blood flowing and warms up the muscles, making them easier to move during the subsequent activity. The second is stretching exercises to increase joint and muscle flexibility.

How will you know when your cardiovascular system is warmed up? After a few minutes of rhythmic movement, your heart rate should be slightly elevated, and you may feel as though you're about to break a sweat. Next, a few stretching exercises should follow—to increase joint and muscle flexibility.

Warm-up exercises should be workout specific. If, for example, you're going to be doing a workout focused on your legs, it's a good idea to get your body ready for that activity by doing some exercises that warm up those muscles and joints.

Each of the exercises below is designed to warm up and stretch the major muscle groups such as the back, chest, shoulders, arms, trunk, and legs. You'll find specific warm-up and cool-down exercises for each of the five workouts recommended at the beginning and end of each exercise routine.

The Cool-down

Like the warm-up, the cool-down consists of two different types of activities: a light intensity rhythmic movement and stretching exercises. The type of cool-down exercises you do after a workout depends on the kind of activities you've been doing.

After a workout where you've been moving continuously, such as the Calorie-Burning Workout or the Aerobic Fitness Workout, do the same kind of rhythmic movements at a slower pace and lighter intensity than during the workout, so that, over several minutes, your body can come to a gentle and comfortable stop. Neglecting this component of your workout can cause you to feel light-headed, as blood tends to settle in exercised muscles and not enough gets back to the heart to be pumped to the brain. The same strategy applies after a walking, dancing, or biking workout—continue the activity, but at a slower pace, for a few minutes before you stop completely.

Five minutes of stretching the muscles you've just exerted should follow. For example, after a walking workout, focus on stretching the muscles of your legs.

When you spend time stretching at the end of a workout, you really notice the benefits! First, it can help to relieve muscle tightness. Second, it's the time when you're most likely to improve your flexibility. You'll notice that warm muscles are more receptive to being stretched, and that, after exercising, your muscles are more supple and flexible than they were during the warm-up. You'll be able to stretch further and more thoroughly, and this can help you improve your flexibility!

Whereas you usually hold a stretch for 15 to 30 seconds, while warming up, hold it a little longer during the cool-down, for 30 seconds to 1 minute. Take your time with these stretches. Remember that holding the stretches a little longer is when flexibility is really increased.

Stretch Right

◆ Stretch slowly to the point where you feel a mild tension (stretching or pulling sensation) develop in your muscles. Hold this position without bouncing for 15 to 30 seconds.

◆ Breathe normally. Don't hold your breath while stretching.

◆ For stretches done from a standing position, fix your eyes on a point in front of you to help maintain balance and proper body alignment.

◆ Relax the rest of your body and concentrate on relaxed breathing as you hold the stretch.

CARDIOVASCULAR WARM-UP

 1 Lift arms up overhead so hands touch. Bring arms down to sides. Repeat without stopping.

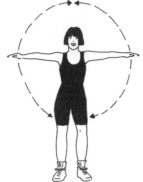

 2 Make wide circles with arms. Circle your arms forward for part of the time, then reverse directions and circle to the back.

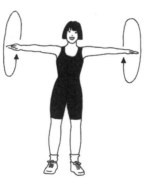

 3 March in place with an exaggerated arm swing.

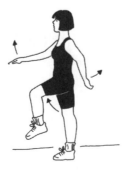

Step sideways with right leg and bring left leg next to right. Step left and repeat. Crisscross arms continuously while you step.

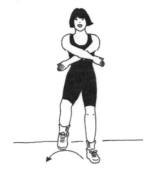

THE WARM-UP/COOL-DOWN STRETCHES

Torso

 Stand and take hold of left wrist with right hand above head. Pull to right. Keep torso stationary as you pull to right. Repeat on other side.

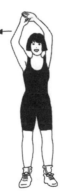

 Stand with back to wall. Turn upper body until you can touch wall with both hands at shoulder level.

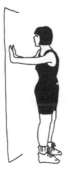

Neck

 Lower right ear toward right shoulder. Repeat on other side.

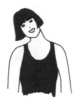

Shoulders

 Place hands behind back and clasp hands together. Lift arms until you feel a stretch. Keep shoulders down and relaxed.

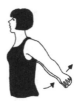

 Place arms overhead and clasp hands together. Push arms back slightly.

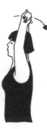

Hip

10 Bend right knee, as shown, placing hands on left thigh to support body weight. Keeping back straight, gently push hips forward until knee is over foot. Repeat with other leg.

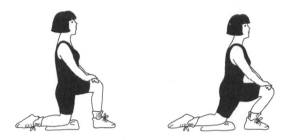

11 Hold onto wall for support. Pull one knee into chest. Slightly bend knee of standing leg. Repeat with other leg.

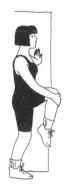

Calf

12 Place one leg in front of the other. Lean on front leg. Extend back leg, keeping heel pressed to floor. Repeat with other leg.

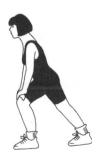

Hold onto wall for support. Place balls of feet on edge of a stair, with heels hanging over edge. Lower heels and hold.

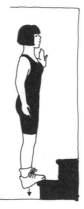

Quadriceps

 Bend left leg behind you and hold that foot with left hand. If you need to, hold onto wall or chair for balance. Repeat with other leg.

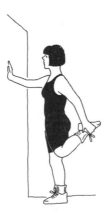

Hamstring

 With one foot elevated, keeping back straight, lean forward over straightened leg. Repeat with other leg.

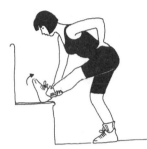

Inner Thigh

 Lie on back. Bend knees and let them drop toward floor. Keep soles of feet together.

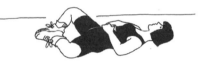

Upper Back

 Stand with knees slightly bent and hands on top of thighs. Keep head up. As you slowly round up lower back and shoulders, drop head. Slowly return to starting position.

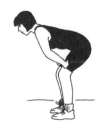 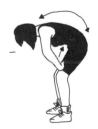

Kneel on floor. Extend arms over head on floor. Press hands to floor.

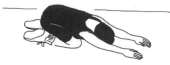

Lower Back

 Lie on floor, arms extended out to either side. Bend knees and lower them to the right. Turn your head and look to the left. Repeat on other side.

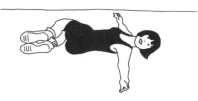

Full Body

 Stand on tiptoe, while extending both arms overhead.

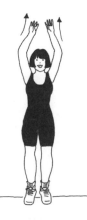

The Right Way to Lift

Picking up a child, lifting heavy boxes, moving furniture—lifting is part of everyday life. Strong and flexible muscles—and proper lifting technique—can help ensure that you don't injure your lower back or experience other musculoskelatal injuries. Keep in mind these important points:

1. Keep feet apart to provide a base of support.
2. Place your hands on the object, and using your leg muscles to power the lift, stand up.
3. Keep the object as close to your body as possible.
4. Keep your back straight as you lift.

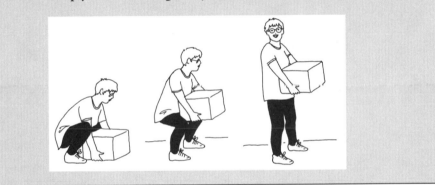

Stretching and Strengthening Your Way to a Healthy Back

Many of us have backs that are often out of whack. When back pain strikes, it's more difficult to move—which means it's harder to stay fit and quite easy to gain a few pounds.

While back problems are sometimes the result of injury or congenital abnormality, many are caused when the body is out of shape. By increasing flexibility in the back and upper legs, and improving muscular strength in the abdomen and back, you'll be on your way to making your back stronger and healthier. Flexibility and strengthening exercises are often recommended for prevention and rehabilitation of low back strain. If you have a history of back problems, be sure to get your physician's approval before doing these, or any other exercises. See exercises on the following page.

The collection of exercises that follows is designed to get your back in shape. These exercises address the common problems of inadequate strength and flexibility mentioned on the previous page. A detailed description of each exercise can be found on the noted pages (see pages 33, 60–63, and 74–77).

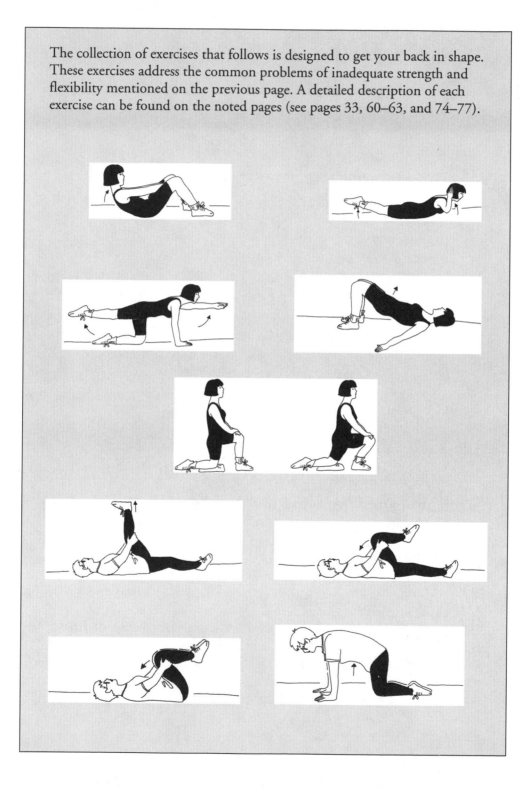

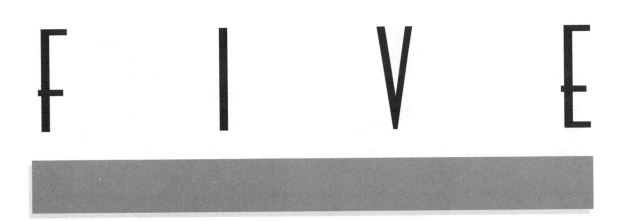

F I V E

Calorie-Burning Workout

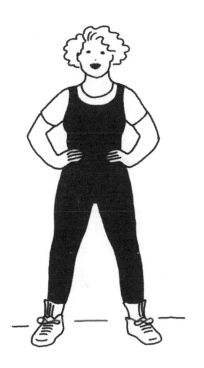

A calorie-burning workout does exactly that—it burns calories! And although all exercise burns calories, calorie-burning workouts are designed to maximize this aspect of exercise. Calorie-burning workouts are composed of movements that rely on the large muscle groups of the body. In these workouts, you burn a significant number of calories, fueling the muscles that are exercised. And, because the intensity of the workout is kept light to moderate, it encourages you to have a longer workout, maximizing the calorie-burning effect.

As you know, your weight is determined by the balance between how much you eat—"calories in"—and how many calories you burn—"calories out." Your body weight remains stable—weight maintenance—when the number of calories contained in the food you eat is balanced by an equal number of calories burned. When the balance between calories in and calories out is disrupted, the result is either weight gain or weight loss.

Eating fewer calories should result in weight loss. However, relying only on eating less food as a means of weight loss is not the most effective way. Long-term weight control can be more comfortable and more effective when you combine eating less with an increase in the number of calories burned, that is, an increase in physical activity.

Lots of daily physical activities help you burn extra calories—walking to do errands, climbing stairs, and doing household chores and yardwork. But there are other effective ways to burn calories such as hiking, walking, biking, jogging, dancing, and swimming. What do these activities have in common? Each one requires the sustained and continuous movement of the large muscle groups. Remember, you burn calories fueling the contraction of these muscles.

What Will a Calorie-Burning Workout Do for Me?

◆ Help me lose weight when exercise is coupled with a reduced-calorie balanced diet.

◆ Promote favorable changes in body composition. The combination of a reduced-calorie diet and increased physical activity results in a greater loss of fat, compared to an equivalent amount of weight lost by a reduced-calorie diet.

◆ Provide a sense of empowerment, control, and improved self-image by allowing me to take charge and make the time to become more active. Over time, this can strengthen my long-term commitment to weight control efforts.

◆ Improve my health and fitness.

Keep in mind, however, that not all recreational activities provide a calorie-burning workout. Playing softball doesn't burn as many calories as biking, for example, because softball involves short bursts of activity, coupled with long periods of inactivity, rather than sustained periods of continuous movement. And when you play golf, it's the sustained periods of walking that make this a good calorie-burning activity—swinging the club does not contribute all that much.

Yes, a Calorie-Burning Workout Can Be Fun

Our Calorie-Burning Workout should feel more like "dancing" than exercising. It's a workout that's done to music (you will find tips on selecting music on page 23), and is meant to be fun. In fact, it's purposefully designed for people who want to exercise and get moving, but don't think they are interested in "exercise"!

Another advantage of the workout is that while you're moving in time to the music, you'll also achieve health benefits. As discussed in Chapter 1, you reap many health benefits doing modest amounts of physical activity on a regular basis. Research shows that the greatest health benefits occur in sedentary people who begin to exercise moderately. The good news is that you don't have to become a slave to exercise in order to benefit.

What's important about this, and any other, calorie-burning workout is having fun, being comfortable, and burning calories. Research indicates that people tend to stick with an exercise program when it's enjoyable, comfortable, and designed to help them reach their goals.

Remember, the calorie-burning effects of exercise are cumulative. For example, it doesn't matter whether you exercise twice a day for 20 minutes, or once a day for 40 minutes—the number of calories burned will be the same. You decide what best fits your schedule—shorter, more frequent workouts or longer, less frequent ones. Provided the intensity and total time spent exercising are similar, you'll burn a similar number of calories. In addition, when it comes to calorie-burning there is no minimal threshold—no minimal amount you must do in order to achieve calorie-burning benefits. Any additional activity you add to your day can help.

Remember that your ability to lose or maintain weight while doing the Calorie-Burning Workout also depends on your *overall* level of physical activity and your diet—that is, the balance between "calories in" and "calories out."

Getting Started

◆ Give yourself time to build up to a 20- to 30-minute workout. Beginners should aim for 5 or 10 minutes of continuous activity, and slowly add on to the workout in increments of 1 to 2 minutes. Don't worry about not doing more. You'll benefit from any amount of calorie-burning activity, and whenever you can add a little extra, do it!

◆ If you're feeling fatigued or having trouble sustaining the workout at any time, take smaller steps and reduce the movement of the arms. Putting your hands on your hips or keeping your arms at your sides will reduce the intensity of your workout.

◆ Keep in mind that it's more beneficial, from a calorie-burning standpoint, to perform the workout for a longer period of time at a reasonable pace than to perform the workout near maximum intensity for a shorter period of time.

How Much/How Often

◆ If your daily schedule permits, you can do the Calorie-Burning Workout for 20 to 30 minutes every day.

◆ If you're like many people and don't have that much time for exercise in your schedule, aim for doing the workout 4 to 5 days a week.

◆ If you can't fit in that much time, do the workout 3 times a week, trying to make your exercise sessions longer whenever you can.

What Body Changes Can I Expect?

Don't expect to see results overnight. But if you stick with the workout and follow a reduced-calorie balanced diet, you should see noticeable changes in your body—for example, looser-fitting clothes, a smaller waist size, weight loss—in several weeks. If you're not following a reduced-calorie diet, yet still eating within reason, doing the Calorie-Burning Workout should help you maintain your current weight level.

Workout Routines

The Calorie-Burning Workout consists of five combinations of four steps—the workout is versatile and easily adjusts to your fitness level and ability.

In determining how long to do the workout, first consider this question: How much time do I have? If you have only 10 minutes, do the workout for that long. Slowly build up to doing the workout for at least 20 to 30 minutes.

◆ If you are a beginner, or you haven't been active for a while, do each step 4 times. Try to do the whole workout, but if you become fatigued, eliminate one or more of the sequences.

◆ If you have been active, and can comfortably complete the whole workout once, repeat the sequences in order from the beginning to complete a 20- to 30-minute workout.

◆ Once you've mastered the workout, be your own choreographer and customize the workout. As you learn some new steps or develop your own, feel free to add them to your routine.

THE CALORIE-BURNING WORKOUT

The Warm-up

Do warm-ups ◆1◆, ◆3◆, and ◆4◆ on pages 30–31 for 2 to 3 minutes, until your heart rate is slightly elevated and you feel as though you're about to break a sweat.

Do stretching exercises for about 5 minutes—stretches ◆5◆, ◆8◆, ◆10◆, ◆12◆, ◆14◆, ◆15◆, ◆16◆, and ◆19◆ (pages 31–36).

If you're not sure what step comes next, march in place for a few seconds—it's a good transition step if you lose your place.

The Workout

 1 Walk forward 4 steps. Touch toe to floor in front and clap. Walk back 4 steps, touch toe behind and clap.

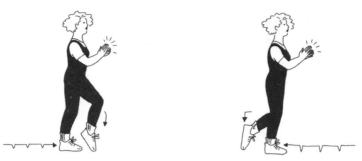

 2 Start with arms extended out to side, elbows slightly bent. Keeping elbows out, bend forearms in so that palms are facing chest. Walk forward and back 4 steps, while moving arms.

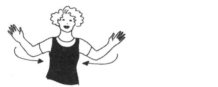

 3 Start with arms in front of you at chest level. Alternate crossing one arm over the other in front of you as you walk forward and back 4 steps.

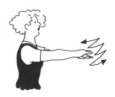

Start with arms at waist. As you walk forward 4 steps, punch arms 4 times, raising them higher each time until they're overhead. Lower arms the same way as you walk back.

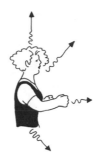

 Start with arms at sides. Kick back with bent knee, alternating legs. At the same time that you kick back, bring forearms up to shoulder. Keep elbows tucked at waist.

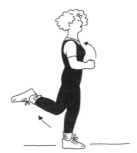

 Keep elbows tucked at waist and extend forearms back each time you kick back.

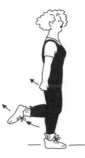

Start with hands at shoulder height. Push arms forward each time you kick back.

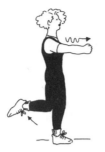

 Start with hands on shoulders. Extend palms toward ceiling each time you kick back.

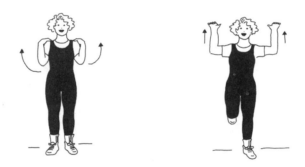

Side-to-Side Step Touch

 Place hands on hips and stand with legs apart, feet pointing straight ahead. Lower your body.

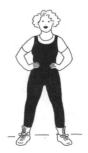 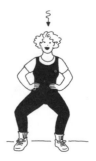

From the same starting position as in the previous exercise, extend leg on one side, touching opposite toe to floor as you shift weight to other leg. Return to starting position. Alternate legs.

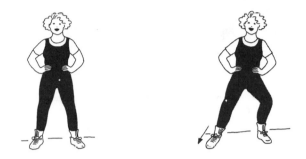

 Extend same side arm as you extend leg. Alternate legs.

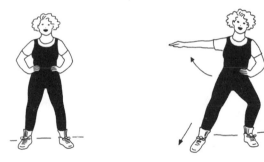

 Extend both arms as you extend leg. Alternate legs.

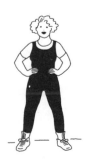 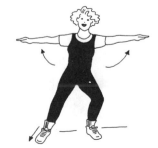

Start with arms overhead. Lift one knee, bringing arms down on either side of lifted knee. Stand straight throughout movement. Alternate legs.

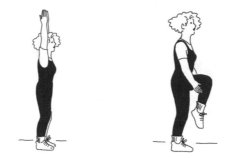

 Start with arms overhead. Lift one leg, with knee slightly bent, bringing opposite arm down to touch leg at shin. Alternate legs.

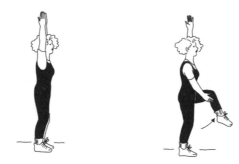

 Lift knee on a diagonal from torso. Bring elbows in and out at waist. Bring elbows in each time you lift knee. Alternate legs.

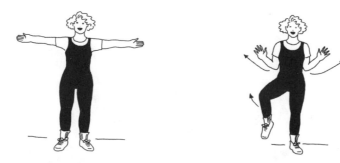

16   Face front. Shuffle to right 4 steps, leading with right shoulder. Repeat to left.

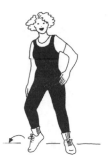

 17   Step sideways with left leg, right leg crosses behind left, step sideways with left, bring right leg next to left. Repeat starting with right leg. Clap twice, during cross-back and when legs are together.

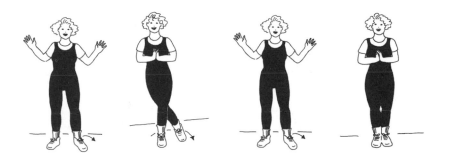

18   Start with hands on shoulders and extend palms toward ceiling during cross-back and when legs are together. Repeat, starting with other leg.

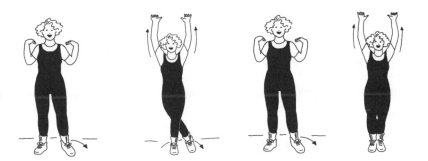

Start with arms out to sides, elbows at shoulder height and bent at 90-degree angles. Bring arms in front of you during cross-back and when legs are together. Repeat, starting with other leg.

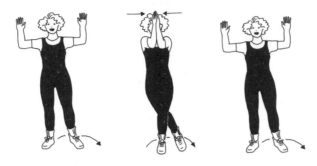

 Stand in modified lunge position, right leg back, left leg bent in front. Right arm is extended back, left arm is bent and in front. Bring right leg in toward chest, bend right arm in toward chest and extend left arm back. Left leg is stationary. Switch legs after completing repetitions on one side.

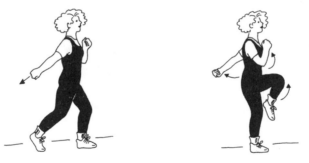

The Cool-down

After a workout in which you've been moving continuously, slow down the pace, before your body comes to a complete stop. Spend a few minutes doing a few of the basic steps you did at the beginning of this workout, at a slower pace and lighter intensity.

Spend about 5 minutes stretching. Remember, after a workout hold each stretch a little longer, about 30 seconds or more. Do stretches **6**, **9**, **11**, **13**, **14**, **15**, **16**, and **20** (pages 31–36).

S I X

Toning and Strengthening Workout

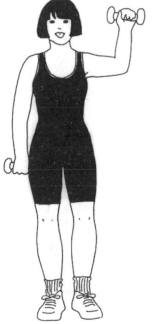

Developing the strength, or force-generating ability, of your muscles is an important part of being fit. Strong muscles are necessary in many of our daily activities—from climbing stairs to lifting groceries to pushing a lawnmower. Strong muscles help improve posture. They also improve your performance in sports and

51

help prevent injury in sports or recreational activities.

Resistance training is based on the principle that your muscles become stronger when you challenge them to work harder than usual. When you do resistance-training exercises on a regular basis, you'll find that, over time, your muscles adapt to the harder work and become stronger, firmer, and more toned. If you complement a strengthening workout with calorie-burning exercise, your muscles develop a firm, lean look as you lose fat and conserve muscle.

The way to challenge muscles is to work against resistance, which can either be the weight of your own body (as in curl-ups or push-ups) or weights such as hand or ankle weights, barbells, elasticized bands, or other

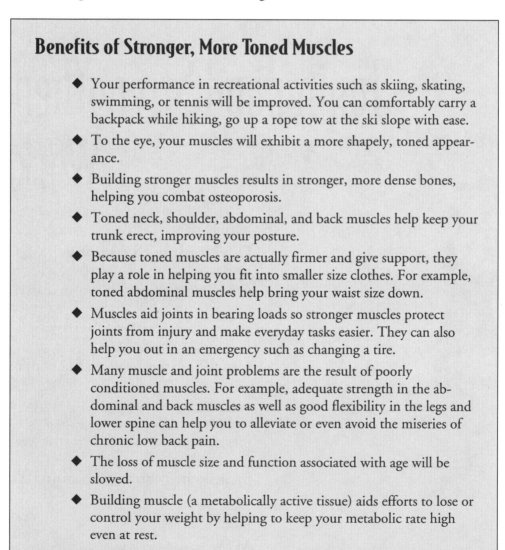

Benefits of Stronger, More Toned Muscles

◆ Your performance in recreational activities such as skiing, skating, swimming, or tennis will be improved. You can comfortably carry a backpack while hiking, go up a rope tow at the ski slope with ease.

◆ To the eye, your muscles will exhibit a more shapely, toned appearance.

◆ Building stronger muscles results in stronger, more dense bones, helping you combat osteoporosis.

◆ Toned neck, shoulder, abdominal, and back muscles help keep your trunk erect, improving your posture.

◆ Because toned muscles are actually firmer and give support, they play a role in helping you fit into smaller size clothes. For example, toned abdominal muscles help bring your waist size down.

◆ Muscles aid joints in bearing loads so stronger muscles protect joints from injury and make everyday tasks easier. They can also help you out in an emergency such as changing a tire.

◆ Many muscle and joint problems are the result of poorly conditioned muscles. For example, adequate strength in the abdominal and back muscles as well as good flexibility in the legs and lower spine can help you to alleviate or even avoid the miseries of chronic low back pain.

◆ The loss of muscle size and function associated with age will be slowed.

◆ Building muscle (a metabolically active tissue) aids efforts to lose or control your weight by helping to keep your metabolic rate high even at rest.

resistance-training equipment. It doesn't matter which type of resistance equipment you choose—your muscles will respond the same way, whether you use barbells, multi-station exercise equipment, or elasticized bands.

The point is to work your muscles at a level that challenges them. This means that the amount of exercise you can do when you start the Toning and Strengthening Workout will not be sufficient to challenge your muscles a few weeks into your exercise program, as you will have become stronger. As you progress, you'll need to either increase the number of times you do each exercise or increase the resistance your muscles work against (for example, lift heavier weights) to challenge your muscles. Once you're satisfied with your strength and muscle tone, it's all right to stay at the level that brought you to that point—that is, amount of weight lifted, repetitions completed, and frequency of workouts—and not continually challenge your muscles.

If you do the workout on a regular basis, you can expect to see results in four to six weeks. At that time, you'll begin to feel stronger and notice that your muscles have become firmer and more toned.

How Often Should I Do the Toning and Strengthening Workout?

Unlike other kinds of exercise that you can do every day, plan to do the Toning and Strengthening Workout about three times a week, every other day. Not

Got Five Spare Minutes? Use Them to Tone Up

Everyone has a "problem spot," an area they would like to tone up or a muscle they would like to be stronger. Commit to using a few five-minute periods throughout the week to attack your problem spot. Convert down time to constructive time; pick an exercise from this chapter that addresses your problem spot. Consider one or more of the following options:

◆ Talking on the phone at home—toe raises for calves or wall squats for thighs
◆ Watching TV—curl-ups for the abdomen or leg raises for the thighs
◆ Stuck in traffic—squeeze and release a tennis ball to improve grip strength

Every little bit helps!

only do you have to challenge your muscles to build strength and tone, but you have to provide them with a rest so that development can take place. If you want to do toning exercises more frequently, you can, as long as you plan on giving the muscles worked a "recuperative" day. For example, you can work the upper body one day, and the lower body the next.

Repetitions and Sets—How Many Should I Do?

Repetitions are the number of times you repeat each exercise. Sets are groups of repetitions performed without stopping or resting.

◆ If you're a beginner, start slowly. Do the "Beginner" modification of each exercise, and aim for doing each exercise 12 times in a row. Stop if you feel pain, are unable to maintain proper form, or if your muscles become fatigued. If you can't do 12 at first, don't be discouraged. Congratulate yourself on the number of repetitions you can do!

◆ When you can comfortably complete 15 to 20 repetitions of an exercise, consider either adding a short rest and another set of the same exercise or moving on to a more challenging exercise for the same group of muscles.

Increasing the Challenge—A Progressive Strategy

Here's an easy-to-follow progressive strategy:
1. Do as many reps as you comfortably can, aiming for 12.
2. Do 15-20 comfortably.
3. When you can do 15 to 20 comfortably—remember, you're working at your own pace, and it may take 2 or 3 weeks—do one of the following:
   ◆ Take a short rest and do another set of the same exercise.
   ◆ Move to next exercise level (for example, from beginner to intermediate) for more challenge.
   ◆ Add resistance (for example, add weight, or more challenging elasticized bands, etc.).
4. When you're again able to complete 15 to 20 repetitions comfortably, it's time to challenge your muscles with one of the above techniques.

◆ A more challenging exercise or an additional set of the same exercise will reduce the number of repetitions you can do, but don't be discouraged! Without this new challenge, your muscles will not become stronger or more toned. You'll notice that, over time, you're able to do 15 to 20 repetitions again. Then it's time to either add more resistance or do an additional set of the exercise. Remember, once you're satisfied with your strength and muscle tone, it's okay to stay at the level where you are, and not continue to challenge your muscles.

Do You Want Muscle Strength or Muscle Tone?

What is your primary goal—building muscle strength or developing muscle tone, the firm lean look of a muscle? Follow these strategies to reach your goal:

The fastest way to build
strong muscles   =   Heavy resistance and low repetitions

The best way to improve muscle
endurance, burn calories, and
give muscles a firm, toned look   =   Light resistance and many repetitions

---

Body Changes—What You Can Expect

You'll definitely notice the changes your body experiences as a result of the Toning and Strengthening Workout.

Don't be alarmed if you feel tightness or soreness in your muscles or joints one or two days after doing the workout. This is to be expected. It's an indication that you exercised little-used muscles or challenged muscles in a new and more vigorous way. (For more information on what feelings to expect when you exercise, see What Exercise Should Feel Like, page 19.)

Don't confuse the Toning and Strengthening Workout with spot reduction, which is the notion that you lose more fat in the area of a specific muscle exercised. There is no evidence that spot reduction works or that you'll necessarily lose fat near exercising muscles. Instead, remember that when you combine exercise with a reduced-calorie balanced diet, you lose fat from all over your body. Toning exercises strengthen muscles and give them a firmer, toned

Equipment ABCs

You can learn all about buying hand-held and ankle weights, and elasticized bands, at your local sporting goods store. Here are some general guidelines to follow:

◆ Hand weights. Hand weights come in a variety of shapes and sizes. Some are designed with a special hand grip, and additional weights can be added to each side, allowing you to adjust the weight to meet your needs.

Solid dumbbells, made of iron, are also popular; they come in a variety of different weights from 1 to 10 pounds. The advantage of solid weights is that they don't have to be put together and you don't have to worry about weights slipping off the ends. The disadvantage: To keep your muscles challenged, you will need to buy heavier weights as your strength improves.

◆ Ankle weights. Ankle weights are often made of leather or vinyl belts and have Velcro-strap closures. They are available with 1- to 5-pound (or 1- to 10-pound) weights for each ankle. You adjust the weight by adding or removing small metal weights from pouches in the belt.

◆ Elasticized bands. Elasticized bands or tubes are like rubber bands, only much larger. They are often color-coded to help differentiate between resistance levels. Be sure to purchase a band that matches your strength level.

appearance, but they don't make specific fat deposits disappear. No exercise program can do that.

As you continue to do the resistance-training workout, your muscles will tone up—they'll actually feel harder. If you progressively challenge your muscles, you'll begin to see muscle definition. There's nothing like visible results to inspire you and help you stick with a workout!

Toning and Strengthening Workout Tips

◆ Keep breathing. Never hold your breath during resistance-training exercises.

◆ Learn proper form. Paying attention to form—where you place your feet, position your neck and back, and the direction in which you look—helps prevent injury and ensures that you're exercising the targeted muscle.

◆ Do each exercise slowly, not relying on gravity or momentum to do the work for you. Moving slowly—and in a controlled way—ensures that the targeted muscle is doing the work.

◆ Fix your eyes on a point in front of you to help maintain balance and proper body position.

◆ Enjoy music during your toning workout. It can be motivating and pleasant, but don't sacrifice form or technique trying to keep the beat.

◆ Stop immediately if you feel pain. Any sharp pain is a warning that you may be overdoing it. The more you exercise, the more you'll learn the difference between how your muscles should feel when you exercise and an acute pain that tells you when you're overdoing it or heading for an injury.

◆ If you're a beginner, and aren't sure whether you've achieved the correct position, use a full-length mirror to ensure that you're doing the move accurately. Or ask someone to watch you and get feedback about your position.

TONING AND STRENGTHENING WORKOUT

The Warm-up

Do warm-ups ❶, ❷, and ❸ (page 30) for 2 to 3 minutes, until your heart rate is slightly elevated and you feel as though you're about to break a sweat.

Do stretching exercises for about 5 minutes: stretches ❺, ❽, ❿, ⓬, ⓯, ⓱, and ⓳ (pages 31–36).

Please note that, for most of the exercises that follow, the intermediate position is illustrated when appropriate. For an easier or more challenging modification of each exercise, look for the heading "Beginner" or "Advanced" under each exercise.

Legs

1 Calf

Stand on a low platform or step with heels extended over the edge. Keep your head erect and back straight and look straight ahead. (You may want to hold onto a wall at waist level for balance.) Lower heels, then lift up on toes into a tip-toe position.

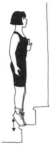

Beginner: Perform same movement standing on the floor, instead of a step.

Advanced: Sit on floor, legs extended in front of you, elasticized band around toes or ball of one foot. Hold band at thighs or higher. Push toes forward, then relax. Repeat with other leg.

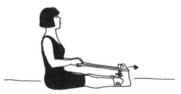

2 Outer Thigh

Stand with back straight, head up, and eyes fixed on object ahead to improve balance. Lift leg to side. Keep knee that is lifted facing forward. Use light ankle weights, or an elasticized band, placing it around ankles and pulling one leg away from the other. Repeat with other leg.

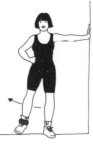

Beginner: Lift leg as shown below, without ankle weights or elasticized bands.

Advanced: Wear heavier ankle weights or use more resistant elasticized band.

Outer Thigh

Lie on one side, bottom knee bent. Slowly lift and lower outer leg. Make sure knee and foot of outer leg face forward, not up. Repeat with other leg.

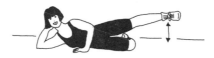

Beginner: Do this exercise standing up, lifting leg out to the side, until you have isolated the appropriate muscle group and can do the move in a slow and controlled manner.

Advanced: Wear ankle weights or use elasticized band. Keeping both legs straight, place band around thighs and pull one leg up and away from the other.

 Inner Thigh

Lie on one side. Cross top leg over lower leg. Lift lower leg as high as you can off floor, keeping foot pointed. Repeat with other leg.

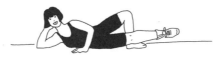

Advanced: Wear ankle weights or place elasticized band on toe of working foot and heel of other leg and perform movement as described above.

 Front Thigh

Sit in hard chair. Lift one foot off floor and extend leg straight in front of you. Repeat with other leg.

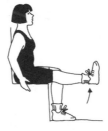

Advanced: Wear ankle weights or place elasticized band around ankle of exercised leg and under other foot. Perform movement as described above.

Buttocks, Back, and Thighs

 Buttocks

Kneel with forearms on floor. Keep back flat, neck relaxed, and head up. Slowly lift bent knee toward ceiling. Concentrate on keeping bottom of foot facing ceiling. Do not lift thigh higher than pictured below. Repeat with other leg.

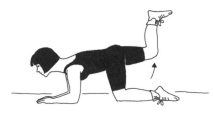

Advanced: Wear ankle weights.

 Buttocks, Back, and Thighs

Lie on back, knees bent, with heels next to buttocks. Slowly lift buttocks and back off floor until thighs and back form a straight line. Hold position for 10–15 seconds.

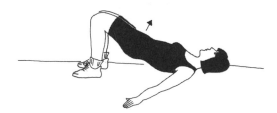

Advanced: Perform exercise as described above. When in up position, extend one leg and hold for 10–15 seconds. Repeat with other leg.

8 **Thighs**

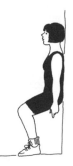

Beginner: Place back flat against wall, arms at sides, heels away from wall. Bend knees while sliding back down wall. Do not bend knees more than 90 degrees. Try to hold body in squat position against wall for 20 seconds at a time or longer. Return to standing.

Advanced: Stand with back to chair, feet parallel, with toes pointing forward. Keeping head up and back straight, bend knees until you are almost sitting in the chair. Return to standing and repeat.

Abdominals

 ### Abdominals

Make a double chin by tucking chin toward chest. Slowly curl head, neck, and shoulders up off floor. Keep arms extended between bent legs, feet flat on floor.

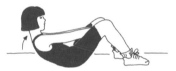

Beginner: Cross arms over chest. Lift head and neck off floor.

Advanced: Cross arms over chest. Curl lower body in toward chest by bringing bent knees into chest. Curl lower body at same time that you curl in upper body.

 ### Side Abdominals

Place hands at side of head without locking hands. Contract abdominal muscles to bring elbow toward opposite knee. Alternate right and left side.

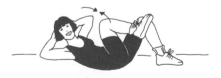

Beginner: Bring knee partway to elbow.

Advanced: Touch elbow to knee.

Side Abdominals

Place left hand at side of head. Bend knees and cross right ankle over left knee. Lift upper body so left elbow approaches right knee. Extend right arm to side.

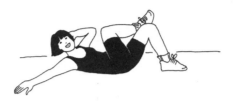

Beginner: Only lift elbow a few inches toward opposite knee.

Advanced: Touch elbow to knee.

Back

Lower Back

Lie on stomach with elbows bent and hands lightly touching ears. Slowly lift head, neck, and chest off floor at same time that you lift feet and legs off floor.

Beginner: Keep arms at side, and lift only head and shoulders.

Advanced: Keep arms extended in front of you as you lift arms, head, neck, chest, feet, and legs off floor.

Back

Kneel on all fours on floor. Slowly lift left arm and right leg at same time. Try to keep both arm and leg parallel to floor.

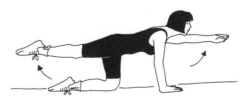

Beginner: Slowly lift left arm. Put it down. Then lift right leg. Put it down. Then lift both arm and leg simultaneously.

Shoulder

 Outer Shoulder

Lift arms to shoulder level. Keep elbows slightly bent. Hold light (1- to 4-pound) hand weights.

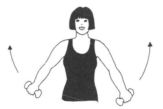

Beginner: When you can do 20 of these comfortably without weights, it's time to add light hand weights.

Advanced: Hold heavier weights.

15 **Top Shoulder**

Place hands at shoulder level, elbows bent, palms facing out. Lift arms over head. Hold light (1- to 4-pound) hand weights.

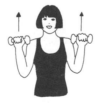

Beginner: When you can do 20 of these comfortably, it's time to add additional light hand weights.

Advanced: Hold heavier weights.

Chest

 Chest Press

Lie on back with knees bent. Lift arms over chest. Hold light (1- to 4-pound) hand weights.

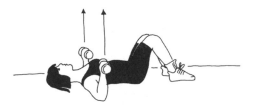

Beginner: When you can do 20 of these comfortably without weights, it's time to add light hand weights.

Advanced: Hold heavier weights.

 Push-ups

Kneel with hands under shoulders. Lower chest to floor, allowing elbows to bend out at sides.

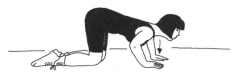

Beginner: Wall push-up. While standing, touch wall with arms extended, elbows slightly bent. Slowly bend arms and lower body toward wall.

Advanced: Modify position illustrated above. Keeping hands under shoulders, move knees back so body is straight from shoulders to knees. From this position, lower chest to floor, allowing elbows to bend out to sides.

Arms

 ### Biceps

Keep elbows close to sides. Bend arms toward shoulders. Hold light (1- to 4-pound) hand weights.

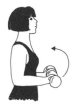

Beginner: If you can do 20 of these comfortably without weights, it's time to add light hand weights.

Advanced: Hold heavier hand weights, or use elasticized band, placing it on one thigh, and pulling up with opposite arm. Place band under one foot and pull up in bicep curl position.

 ### Triceps

Place bent arm behind head. Extend arm over head and return to start position. Hold light (1- to 4-pound) hand weight.

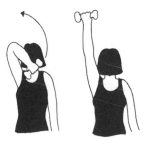

Beginner: When you can do 20 of these comfortably without weights, it's time to add light hand weights.

Advanced: Hold heavier hand weights, or use elasticized band, holding it in support hand and pulling away.

Triceps

Stand with left leg in front of right. Back straight, head erect, eyes looking straight ahead. Lean on left leg. Extend right forearm up and backward, and then bring it back in toward waist. Keep elbow high. Use light (1- to 4-pound) hand weights. Switch legs and repeat on other side.

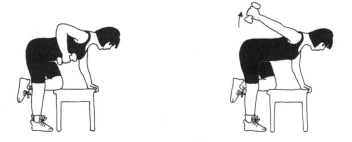

Beginner: When you can do 20 of these comfortably without weights, it's time to add light hand weights.

Advanced: Hold heavier hand weights, or use elasticized band. Place right arm across front of body at waist and hold band. Pull back with left forearm.

The Cool-down

Spend about 5 minutes stretching. Remember, after a workout you should hold each stretch a little longer, about 30 seconds to 1 minute. Do stretches ◆6◆, ◆7◆, ◆9◆, ◆10◆, ◆13◆, ◆15◆, ◆18◆, and ◆19◆ (pages 31–36).

S E V E N

The Flexibility and Stress-Reduction Workout

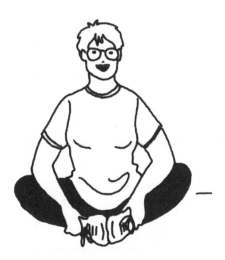

What does it mean to be flexible? It means that your muscles, tendons, and joints are supple and loose. It means that you can move your joints through their full range of motion without stress, injury, or pain.

Each person's flexibility is different. Genetics plays a role; some people are just born more flexible than others. You may even notice that, within your own body, some joints are more flexible than others. For example, your upper body may be tight while your legs and hips are loose and flexible.

The good news is that by doing stretching exercises regularly, you can increase your flexibility. After you've done the Flexibility and Stress-Reduction Workout for several weeks, you'll begin to notice that you can stretch further and with more ease than when you first began. You may even notice improvement after doing the workout just a few times.

As anyone who has ever done yoga can tell you, there are many benefits to making stretching a regular part of your fitness regimen. First, stretching helps limber up your muscles for all other kinds of exercise and sports. Flexible joints and supple muscles are less prone to injury; they perform any movement more easily, cutting down on the chance of muscle strain and soreness.

Stretch Anywhere, Anytime

Driving, operating a computer, or talking on the phone are all activities that can cause muscles and joints to tighten up. A bonus about stretching: You can do it almost anywhere—which means that you can limber up muscles, loosen up joints, and reduce muscle tension throughout the day, without going to the gym or changing into exercise clothes. These get-the-kinks-out stretches are a great addition to this stretching workout.

On-the-Go Stretching Tips

◆ While walking down the hall in the office or at home, do arm raises to rear (stretch 5, page 73), hands above head stretch (stretch 6, page 74), or elbow across chest stretch (stretch 8, page 74).

◆ While standing waiting for a bus or a train, find a curb or step and stretch your calf by alternately placing the heel of each foot off the curb and slowly lowering it toward the ground until you feel tension develop in your calf. (See calf stretch, page 34.)

◆ While standing in line, you can also stretch your leg to the side or to the front, pointing your toe to modify the stretch.

◆ While you're at your desk, do a few neck stretches, shoulder shrugs, or shoulder rolls (stretches 1, 2, 3, and 4, pages 72–73).

Stretching also feels good. The process of stretching is relaxing, peaceful, and calming. When you focus on and stretch specific muscles, it heightens your awareness of how those muscles feel. You'll notice that on some days, tightness in your body is often in direct response to a prolonged period of inactivity, such as long-distance driving or flying. Tight muscles and decreased flexibility are often the result of an inactive lifestyle in which muscles are underused. In addition, certain repetitive or strenuous activities, such as jogging or heavy lifting, can also result in tight muscles.

Once you're able to recognize the feel of "tension," you'll have a better chance of learning how to release it. The Flexibility and Stress-Reduction Workout is designed to help you release excess muscle tension and improve overall flexibility. You can use it to help you relax and relieve tension brought on by everyday stress or incorporate parts of it into a cool-down following your favorite recreational activity. Doing stretching exercises on a regular basis can also give you a tangible sense of accomplishment as you find yourself more and more able to bend, flex, and extend farther than you did before.

Perfecting Your Stretching Technique

To stretch your muscles effectively and improve flexibility, it's important to learn how to stretch properly. If you don't, you could do your body more harm than good. There are correct and incorrect ways to stretch. The safest, most effective way is to stretch and "hold," rather than bounce up and down.

Assume the proper position. Stretch the muscle slightly by holding—not forcing—it. You should feel a little bit of tension (a stretching or pulling sensation) in the muscle; continue to hold the position, and that feeling of tension should ease up and you'll feel the muscle relax. As your muscles and joints respond to the exercise, you'll find that, after the tension of the first stretch subsides, you'll be able to stretch a bit further, again holding the muscle in a lengthened position when you repeat the stretch.

If you feel a sharp pain, or undue discomfort, stop immediately. You're stretching too far if anything hurts.

As with any other kind of exercise, it's important to use proper form. You'll limit your chances of injury and get the full benefit of each stretch.

Stretching Tips

- Do the workout at least three times a week.

- Hold each stretch for 15 to 30 seconds, without bouncing.

- If a particular muscle feels tight, repeat the exercise that stretches that muscle a few more times.

- To maximize your flexibility, increase the time you hold each stretch. Aim for 1 minute for each stretch. You can also do more repetitions of each exercise, or increase the number of days you do the workout.

Stretching Do's

- Focus your attention on the muscles being stretched. This will improve the feeling of relaxation and the overall effects of the stretch.

- Stretch slowly to the point where you feel a mild tension (stretching or pulling sensation) develop in your muscles. Hold this position without bouncing for 15 to 30 seconds.

- Breathe normally. Don't hold your breath while stretching.

- Relax the rest of your body and concentrate on relaxed breathing as you hold the stretch.

- For stretches done from a standing position, fix your eyes on a point in front of you to help maintain balance and proper body position.

- If you're a beginner, and aren't sure whether you've achieved the correct position, use a full-length mirror to ensure that you're doing the move accurately. Or ask someone to watch you and get feedback about your position.

The Five Starter Stretches

If you haven't exercised in a while, and want to gradually incorporate stretching into your life, start by concentrating on these five basic exercises. Try to make them part of your morning ritual by doing them every day before breakfast. After many hours of sleep (inactivity), muscles and joints are often tight. Stretching is a good way to wake up and get moving in the morning. When you find out how good it feels, you may even want to add more stretches to your morning routine.

The Five Starter Stretches are:

◆ Stretch arms above and behind head

◆ Raise arms to rear

◆ Legs toward chest

◆ Kneeling with arms overhead, press palms to floor

◆ Whole body stretch

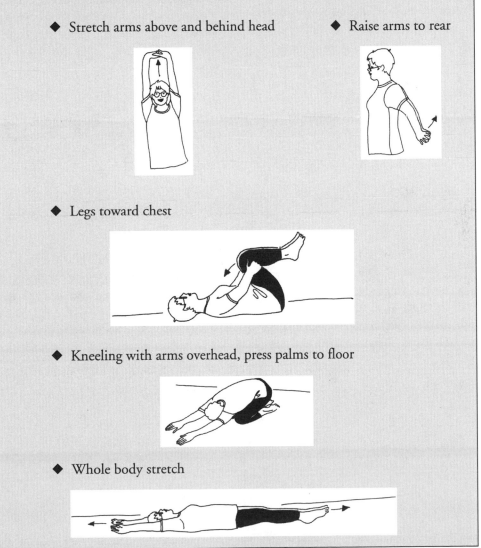

FLEXIBILITY AND STRESS-REDUCTION WORKOUT

Please note that there are two types of flexibility exercises in the workout that follows. Some exercises put your muscles and joints through their range of motion, which helps to relax and loosen them up. Other exercises require holding the position, and involve stretching muscles in order to more effectively develop flexibility.

The Warm-up

Your muscles and joints are easier to stretch, and can be stretched more effectively, when they've been properly warmed up. To warm up before this stretching workout, warm up a little longer than usual. Spend about 5 minutes doing some activities to warm up your muscles and joints. Use warm-ups ◆1, ◆2, ◆3, and ◆4 (pages 30–31), as well as some basic aerobic and dance steps found on pages 102–104.

Neck

1 Turn head to right so you're looking out over right shoulder. Repeat on other side.

2 Keeping torso erect, lift head up so you're looking at ceiling, and down, bringing chin to chest.

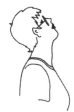

Shoulders

3 Arms at sides. Lift shoulders up toward ears and back down in shrugging motion.

4 Slowly roll shoulders forward in a continuous motion. Repeat, rolling shoulders backward.

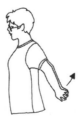

Arms and Shoulders

(Note: The following four stretches can be done standing as well as seated.)

5 Place arms behind back and clasp hands together. Lift arms as shown. Keep shoulders down and relaxed.

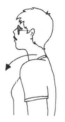

Place arms overhead and clasp hands together. Push arms up and back slightly.

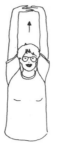

 Raise right arm over head, pointing elbow to ceiling. Grasp right elbow with left hand and pull arm toward left. Repeat on other side.

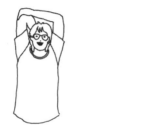 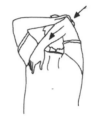

 Grasp elbow as shown, and pull to opposite shoulder. Repeat on other side.

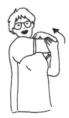

Legs and Feet

 Lying on back, gently pull right knee toward chest and attempt to straighten leg, pushing sole of foot toward ceiling. Repeat with other leg.

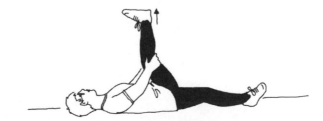

Sit in hard chair. Cross right leg over left and slowly rotate ankle in complete circle. Repeat with other leg.

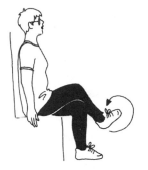

 Sit in hard chair. Cross right leg over left and slowly point toe to floor and hold, then pull toes toward shin and hold. Repeat with other leg.

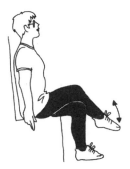

 Lie on left side as shown below. Holding right foot with right hand, pull in toward buttock. Repeat on other side.

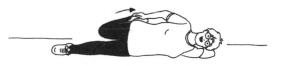

 Sit on floor with soles of feet pressed together. Hold ankles and gently push knees to floor.

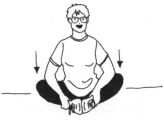

Sit on floor. Cradle left leg in arms and gently pull in toward chest. Repeat with other leg.

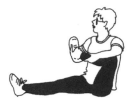

 From a standing position, take one large step forward with your right foot. Keep your left leg straight while you flex your right knee until both hands are low enough to touch the ground. Don't let your right knee extend over your foot.

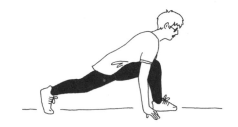

Back

 Lying on back, lift right knee toward chest. Place both hands behind knee and gently pull in toward chest, keeping back flat to floor. Repeat on other side.

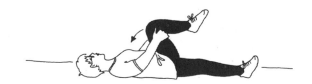

 Lie on floor. Keeping knees together, use hands to bring both knees up and gently pull to chest while keeping back flattened to floor.

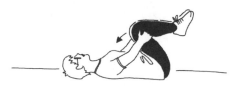

18 Kneel on all fours, keeping back flat. Pull in abdominals, and as you do, arch back upwards. Lower until back is flat, then arch downward.

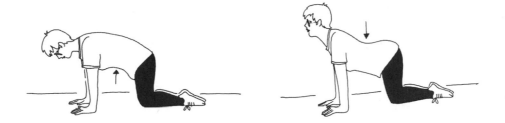

19 Lie on back. Cross bent left knee over extended right leg. Press knee of bent leg with right hand until you feel the stretch in lower back. Make sure shoulders remain on floor. Repeat on other side.

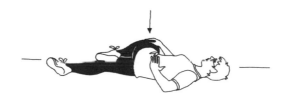

20 Lie on back and bend knees. Place right leg over left and allow left leg to be gently pulled down by right. Repeat on other side.

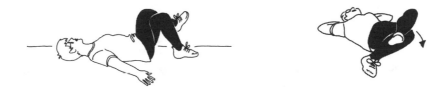

21 Sit on floor, left leg extended, right leg crossed over left. Turn upper body and head to right. Press left arm against right thigh to increase stretch. Repeat on other side.

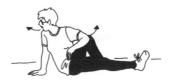

Lie on back, arms extended over head. Stretch arms overhead and lengthen legs so toes are pulling away from body. Feel stretch in upper body, abdominals, and legs.

Reducing Stress

The following stress-reduction technique can be done following the stretching workout. It can also be done following a more vigorous aerobic or calorie-burning workout, or on its own, after a busy day to help you relax.

A word about stress: Because stress is so much a part of our lives, we need ways to control and reduce it. As explained in Chapter 1, regular exercise counters the effects of stress. After physical activity, your body feels more relaxed and so should your mind.

You should feel the tension in your muscles ease after doing the stretching exercises in the Flexibility and Stress-Reduction Workout. But to achieve that relaxed state through more direct action, try the exercise described below.

This stress-reduction technique is specially designed to help people relax. All you need is a few minutes in a quiet place in your home. Once you learn how to do it, you'll be better equipped to handle the stress in your life. Stress-reduction techniques, such as this one, have also proven to be effective in both reducing muscle tension and high blood pressure.

Stress-Reduction Exercise

Sit in a comfortable chair in a quiet room (don't lie down, you may fall asleep.) Close your eyes. To keep your mind from wandering, pay attention to your breathing. Concentrate either on the rise and fall of your stomach, or the inhalation and exhalation of your breath.

Try to stay focused on your breathing and relax your muscles from head to toe. When your mind wanders, bring it gently back to your breathing. Enjoy the peacefulness of the time spent relaxing. Aim for 5 to 10 minutes of relaxation. When finished, slowly count from 1 to 10 and open your eyes. Let yourself recover gradually. Don't stand up suddenly, you may become dizzy. Instead, move your arms around a bit, extend your legs, etc.

As you become more skilled at relaxing, you may want to add a few more minutes to the exercise.

Modification to the technique: Some people prefer to repeat a sound or a word, instead of concentrating on breathing.

E I G H T

Aerobic Fitness Workout

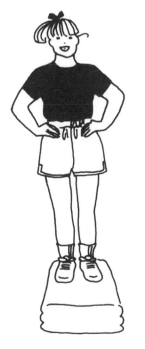

Aerobic fitness, also known as cardiovascular fitness, calls upon your cardiovascular system to deliver oxygen to exercising muscles. Just like calorie-burning workouts, aerobic workouts burn significant calories. And regular aerobic exercise is good for your health.

It can:

- ◆ Reduce body fat.
- ◆ Decrease risk for developing adult-onset diabetes.
- ◆ Strengthen bones.
- ◆ Lessen the risk for certain cancers.
- ◆ Improve your cholesterol profile and blood pressure.
- ◆ Increase your heart's ability to pump blood.

Whereas calorie-burning workouts are performed at a light-to-moderate-intensity level, aerobic fitness workouts require a slightly higher intensity level. That's because you don't condition the cardiovascular system unless you raise your heart rate above its usual level for at least 20 to 30 minutes. Physiologists call this more strenuous exercise "overload."

Your heart rate (expressed in beats per minute) is easily determined by taking your pulse. You can get an accurate count at the side of the neck (place the thumb on the chin and *gently* press the side of your neck with your index and middle fingers). Or place your index and middle fingers on the thumb side of the wrist.

Using a stopwatch or a watch with a second hand, count the number of pulses (heartbeats) in 10 seconds and multiply by 6. That number will indicate your heart rate in beats per minute.

Ways of the Heart (in Aerobic Exercise)

When you exercise to improve aerobic fitness, the goal is to increase your heart rate gradually from resting level, elevate it for a period of time, and then gradually allow it to return to resting level (see graph on page 83).

Warming up, or starting the workout slowly, is extremely important. It ensures that you don't suddenly jolt muscles or put excessive demand on your cardiovascular system. Similarly, at the end of the workout, slowing down, or cooling down, before stopping is also essential. Stopping intense movement abruptly can make you feel dizzy and lightheaded. This happens because blood tends to settle or pool in the previously exercised muscles and not enough gets back to the heart, to be pumped to the brain.

The central part of the workout, its longest segment, is also significant; it's when your heart rate should be elevated and in your target zone. It's during this period of time, when you're exercising in your target zone, that you condition your cardiovascular system.

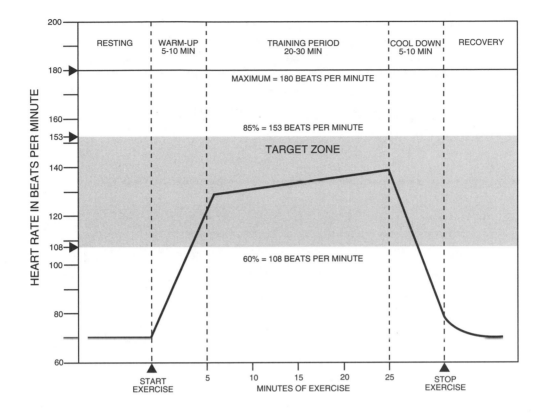

Determining Target Heart Rate

You know how often your heart beats when you're at rest. But just how hard can it work? And more important, how hard does it need to work in order for you to reap the benefits of an aerobic workout?

The highest heart rate attainable with all-out effort is called maximum heart rate. It's estimated by this equation: 220 minus your age in years. For example, a 40-year-old woman's estimated maximum heart rate is 180 beats per minute. To achieve the benefits of aerobic exercise, however, she doesn't have to work at such a high intensity level. Research shows that conditioning of the aerobic system occurs when the heart works at between 60 percent and 85 percent of its maximum rate. A 40-year-old woman's target zone would be 108 beats per minute (60 percent of maximum) to 153 beats per minute (85 percent of maximum). To determine your heart rate, based on age, see the Target Heart Rate Chart on the following page.

If you're just starting out or you haven't exercised in a while, there's nothing wrong with easing into aerobic exercise and working out toward the lower end of the training zone, at 60 percent of maximum. Your body will still reap training benefits. As you do this workout regularly, you'll begin to know how your body feels when you're in the target zone. You'll recognize how much effort it takes to get there, and what your breathing feels like when you're exercising in the target zone. At this point, you may not need to take your pulse, since you'll know by the sensations in your body that you're exercising at the right intensity level.

Target Heart Rate Chart

| | Target Zone | |
Your Age (Years)	*Lower Limit* Heart Rate in Beats/Minute (60%)	*Upper Limit* Heart Rate in Beats/Minute (85%)
20	132	170
25	117	166
30	114	162
35	111	157
40	108	153
45	105	149
50	102	145
55	99	140
60	96	136
65	93	132

For ages not listed above, calculate the upper and lower limits of your target zone by inserting your age and completing the calculations which follow:

A. 220 – Your Age = Age Predicted Maximal Heart Rate

B. Age Predicted Maximal Heart Rate × .60 = Lower Limit

C. Age Predicted Maximal Heart Rate × .85 = Upper Limit

If you're accustomed to using the Rate Your Activity Chart (page 18 in Chapter 3) to determine how hard you're working, continue to do so. When you rate the activity "Somewhat Hard," you are probably working at around 70 percent of maximum heart rate.

How Often Should I Do the Workout?

In determining how often to do an aerobic fitness workout, think about your goals:

1. To maximize your aerobic fitness, do the workout at least 3 days a week, keeping your heart rate in your target zone for about 20 to 30 minutes.

2. To maximize the calorie-burning effect of this work out, do the workout as often as you like (yes, 7 days a week is fine), for about 45 minutes to an hour, at a lower intensity level (maybe 60 percent of maximum heart rate). Exercising for a longer time at the lower end of your target zone provides similar benefits to working out at a higher intensity level for a shorter time.

When Will I See Results?

Your body will begin to adapt to an aerobic workout after about 3 to 4 weeks of regular workouts. It's important to be consistent, however. Just doing the workout once a week won't give you the same benefits as 3 or more times a week.

Here are some changes you may notice:

◆ Able to walk up stairs and do other vigorous activities without panting

◆ Looser-fitting clothing as you lose weight

◆ Able to sustain sports and recreational activities for longer periods of time without undue fatigue

How to Keep Challenging Yourself as Your Aerobic Fitness Improves

The more you do aerobic exercise, the more efficient your cardiovascular system will become. This means you'll be able to tolerate more challenging workouts comfortably, do longer workouts, work out at a higher intensity level, or do more workouts a week.

How will you be able to tell when you're ready to challenge yourself? Once the workout becomes less difficult for you, it's time to up the pace. Use the Rate Your Activity Chart (page 18) as a guideline: if you've been working at a pace you rate as "Somewhat Hard" for weeks, and you now rate the same pace "Fairly Light," it may be time to make your workout more challenging. Similarly, if it takes you longer to reach the point where you notice an increase in your breathing, you are becoming more fit. It may be time to increase the intensity, length, or frequency of your workouts.

Step Training—A Giant Step Toward Better Fitness

Step aerobics is the newest kind of aerobic dance. It combines elements of aerobic dance and working against gravity as you lift and lower your body weight on and off the step. The workout is usually performed to music, and involves a variety of upper and lower body movements.

Step aerobics involves balance and coordination, as well as a degree of strength and cardiovascular conditioning. In addition, step aerobics burns calories while it strengthens and tones the legs and buttocks. The following Step Aerobic Workout is designed to be low impact (one foot is always in contact with the floor or the step), which is easier on your feet and weight-bearing joints than exercise such as high-impact aerobics or jogging.

If you've never exercised on a step, take time to acquaint yourself with it. It may take a little practice before you feel balanced and comfortable stepping up and down on it. When you're accustomed to the feel of the step at a slower pace, practice some of the moves that don't involve the arms. Once you've gained some confidence, it's easy to pick up speed and add arm movements.

Step aerobics grows as you do. Once you've mastered the moves and become more fit, you can increase the intensity of your workout by raising the height of the step.

Workout Routines

The Aerobic Fitness Workout consists of five combinations of four steps; each combination has similar leg movements. The combinations make the workout versatile and easy to adapt to your fitness ability.

In determining how long to do the workout, ask youself: How much time do I have? If you have only 10 minutes, do the workout for that long; then slowly build up to doing the workout for 20 to 30 minutes.

◆ If you are a beginner, or you haven't been active for a while, do each step 4 times. Try to do the whole workout. If you become fatigued, eliminate one or more of the sequences.

◆ If you have been active, and can comfortably complete the whole workout once, repeat the sequences in order from the beginning to fill your 20- to 30-minute workout.

◆ Once you've mastered the workout, be your own choreographer and customize the workout. As you learn some new steps or develop your own, feel free to add them to your routine.

Selecting the Height That's Right For You

Step aerobics can easily be done at home, using one of the many step platforms on the market. These long, vertical platforms are easy to use, and easy to store when not in use. Make sure to purchase a platform that allows you to adjust the height to keep your workouts challenging as your fitness improves.

Choose a height between 4 inches and 12 inches, using these guidelines:

4 to 6 inches for beginners

8 inches for intermediates

10 inches for advanced steppers

12-inch step for well-trained athletes

Step-Right Tips

◆ Make sure you use a step height that's right for you. For example, use a 4-to-6-inch step if you're just starting the workout. (Use the guidelines above to help you find the step height that suits your fitness level.)

◆ Make sure your entire foot fits on the step.

◆ Always step to the center of the step.

◆ Fix your eyes on a point in front of you to help maintain balance and body position. But be sure to glance down at the step every once in a while to check your foot placement.

◆ Stand with your head tall and your back straight when performing these moves.

◆ Never step forward off the step, or jump, hop, or bounce down.

THE STEP AEROBIC WORKOUT

The Warm-up

Do warm-ups ◆2◆, ◆3◆, and ◆4◆ (pages 30–31) for 2 to 3 minutes, until your heart rate is slightly elevated and you feel as though you're about to break a sweat.

Do stretching exercises for about 5 minutes: stretches ◆5◆, ◆7◆, ◆9◆, ◆11◆, ◆13◆, ◆14◆, ◆15◆, and ◆17◆ (pages 31–35).

If you're not sure what step comes next, march in place for a few seconds (it's a good transition step if you lose your place).

Basic

1 Stand facing step, hands on hips. Right foot steps up. Left foot steps up so you're standing on step. Right foot steps down. Left foot steps down so you are in the starting position. Continue on right side, then reverse footwork and step up on left foot.

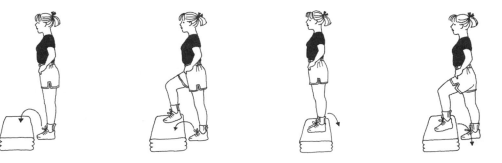

2 To smoothly alternate starting with left and right foot, add the tap. Stand facing step, hands on hips. Right foot steps up. Left foot steps up. Right foot steps down. Toes of left foot tap down on floor and then left foot steps up. Using tap, alternate starting leg each time.

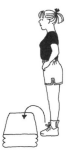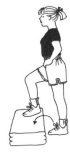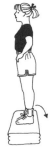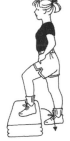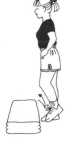

Stand facing step, arms bent, elbows at waist. As right foot steps up, curl arms up toward shoulders. As left foot steps up, arms go back to start position. As you step down with left foot, arms come up again.

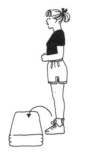 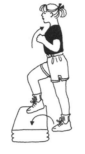 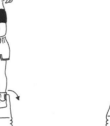 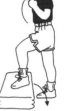

Stand facing step, hands at shoulder height. As right foot steps up, extend forearms overhead. As left foot comes up, arms go back to start position. Right foot steps down, and arms extend back again.

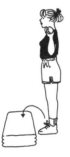 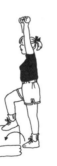 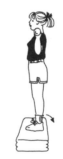 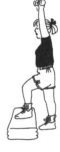

Knee Up

Stand facing step, hands on hips. Right foot steps up. Left foot steps up with lifted knee extended out over step. Left foot steps down. Right foot steps down. Left foot steps up. Right foot steps up with lifted knee.

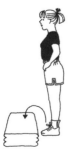 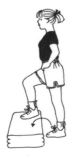 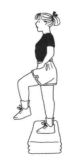 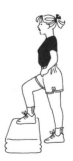

6 Stand facing step, arms bent at sides. As right foot steps up, arms extend out at sides. When left leg lifts up, elbows come into sides. As left foot steps down, arms extend at sides. Right foot steps down and elbows come in.

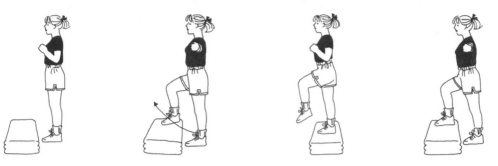

7 Stand facing step, hands on hips. As right foot steps up, extend arms, bending elbows at 90-degree angle at shoulder height. As left leg lifts up, bring arms together in front of chest. As left foot steps down, extend arms. Right foot steps down and arms come together.

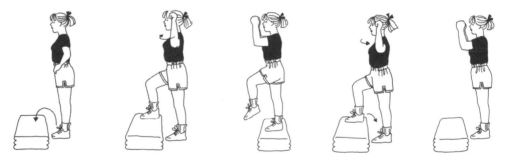

8 Stand facing step, arms bent at sides. As right foot steps up, extend arms overhead. As left leg lifts up, bring arms down on either side of leg. Left foot steps down and arms extend over head. Right foot steps down and arms come down at sides.

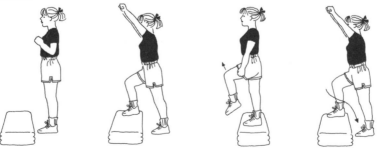

Step Over

 9 Stand with step to your left, hands on hips. Left foot steps up to far side of step, allowing room for right foot. Right steps up and next to left so you're standing sideways on step. Left foot steps down on other side of step, again leaving room for right foot. Right foot taps down next to left and then steps to far side of step, leaving room for left foot.

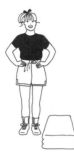 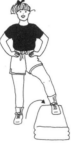 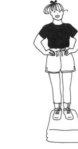 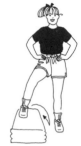

10 Stand with step to your left, hands on hips. As left foot steps up, push arms forward. As right foot steps up, pull elbows back. Then, as left foot steps down push arms forward. Continue to push arms forward and back as you step.

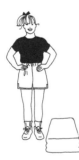 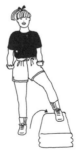 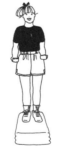 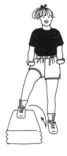

11 Stand with step to your left, arms bent, elbows at sides. As left foot steps up, raise arms at sides to chest height. As right foot steps up, lower arms to start position. Continue to lift and lower arms each time you step.

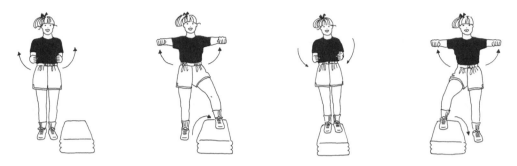

12 Stand with step to your left, arms hanging in front of thighs. As left foot steps up, bring arms up so that backs of hands are almost under chin. Lower arms to start position as right foot steps up. Continue to lift and lower arms each time you step.

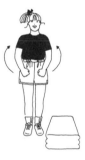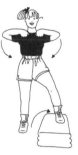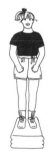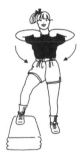

Straddle Up

13 Stand on top of step, facing one end, hands on hips. Left foot steps down, close to left side of step. Right foot steps down close to right side of step so you're straddling step. Left foot steps up. Right foot steps up. Repeat from start position.

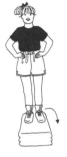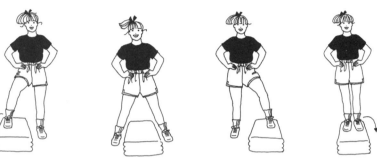

14 Stand on top of step, facing one end, elbows bent and palms facing out from chest. As left foot steps down, push arms out from chest. Bring arms in as right foot steps down. Push arms out as left foot steps up.

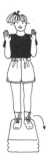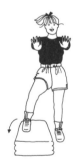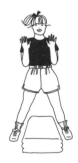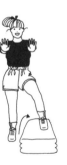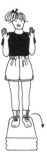

15 Stand on top of step, facing one end, arms out straight in front of you. As left foot steps down, crisscross one arm over the other. Continue to crisscross each time you step.

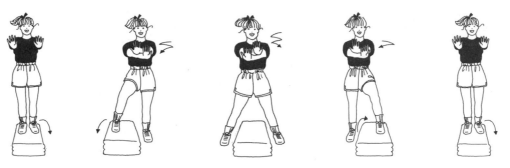

16 Stand in straddle position, legs on either side of step, hands on hips. Left foot steps up. Right foot steps up and knee lifts, then right foot steps down to floor. Left foot steps down. In straddle position, repeat with right foot step up, left foot step up and knee lift. Continue to alternate starting leg.

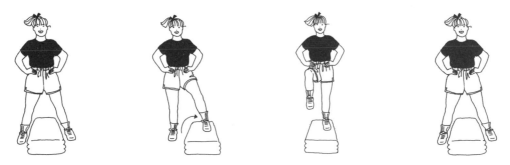

Lunge

17 Stand on top of step, facing one end, hands on hips. Flex right knee and extend left leg back, placing toes on floor. Bring left leg back onto step. Lunge back with right leg.

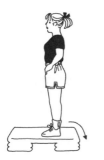 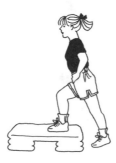 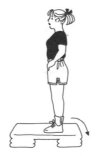 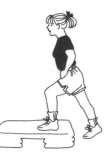

18   Stand on top of step, facing one end, hands on hips. Flex right knee and extend left leg back, punching left arm forward. Bring left leg back onto step. Lunge back with right leg, and punch right arm forward.

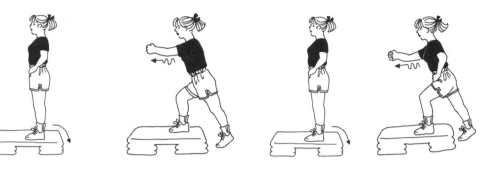

 19   Stand on top of step, facing one end, hands on hips. Flex right knee and extend left leg back, punching arms forward. Bring left leg back onto step. Lunge back with right leg, and punch arms forward.

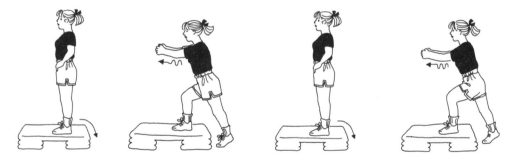

 20   Stand on top of step, facing one end, hands on hips. Flex right knee and extend left leg back, raising left arm in air. Bring left leg back onto step. Lunge back with right leg, and raise right arm in air.

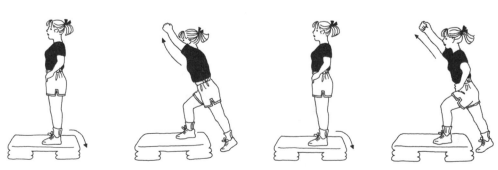

The Cool-down

After a workout where you've been moving continuously, slow down the pace, before your body comes to a complete stop. Spend a few minutes doing a few of the basic steps you did at the beginning of this workout at a slower pace and lighter intensity.

Spend about 5 minutes stretching. Remember, after a workout you're able to hold each stretch a little longer, about 30 seconds or more. Do stretches ◆6, ◆8, ◆10, ◆12, ◆14, ◆15, ◆18, and ◆20 (pages 31–36).

N I N E

Overall Fitness Workout

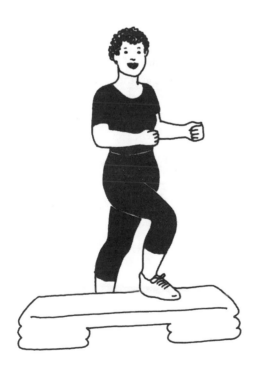

The Overall Fitness Workout is a total body workout that encompasses all the components of the previous workouts: stretching, aerobic activities (providing aerobic fitness and calorie-burning benefits), and muscle toning and strengthening. It's a workout that exercises major areas of the body, and relies on each component of fitness.

99

Each of the other workouts in this book helped you reach one specific fitness goal; the Overall Fitness Workout serves two purposes. It can be used by individuals already in good shape who want to maintain their level of fitness, or by individuals trying to become fit who have not expressed one specific fitness preference.

You may find that the Overall Fitness Workout is similar to exercise videos or exercise classes at the gym. That's because most total body workouts are designed in a comparable way, with a section for warm-up, calorie-burning or aerobic activity, toning and strengthening, a cool-down, and stretching exercises.

Because the Overall Fitness Workout is a total body workout and doesn't put undue stress on any one part of the body, you can do the workout as often as you like during the week. If you do the workout daily, remember to alternate the toning exercises, doing upper body strengthening exercise one day, and lower body exercises the next, to allow your muscles a "recuperative" day.

Workout Routines

The Overall Fitness Workout consists of aerobic dance, step aerobics, and muscle-toning exercises with appropriate warm-up and cool-down segments.

◆ If you are a beginner, or just starting the Overall Fitness Workout, do each aerobic step 4 times. Try to do the whole workout. If you become fatigued, eliminate one or more of the combinations. Remember that step aerobics is generally more vigorous than regular aerobic dance. If you have not been active for some time, consider reducing the number of step aerobic exercises from your routine.

◆ If you are already active, and can comfortably complete the whole work-out, feel free to modify the workout to address your fitness goals as out-lined below.

Here are some suggestions for adapting this versatile workout to your specific needs:

To maximize the calorie-burning effect of the workout:

◆ Do the workout 4 or more days a week.

◆ Repeat the aerobic activity sequence, making the workout longer.

◆ Add additional step aerobics or aerobic dance steps to the workout.

To maximize the cardiovascular effect of the workout:

◆ Do the workout a minimum of 3 days per week.

◆ Concentrate on keeping your heart rate in your target zone throughout the middle portion of the workout.

To maximize the toning and strengthening workout:

◆ Do more repetitions of the Toning and Strengthening exercises.

◆ Add additional exercises from the Toning and Strengthening Workout that address your problem areas.

◆ Work against a resistance (such as weights or elasticized bands) when doing the Toning and Strengthening exercises.

To get more flexibility from the Overall Fitness Workout:

◆ Hold each stretch for a longer period of time, up to 1 minute.

◆ Add additional exercises from the Flexibility and Stress-Reduction Workout that address your problem areas.

THE OVERALL FITNESS WORKOUT

The Warm-up

Do moves ◆1◆, ◆2◆, and ◆3◆ (page 30) for 2 to 3 minutes, until your heart rate is slightly elevated and you feel as though you're about to break a sweat.

Do stretching exercises for about 5 minutes: moves ◆5◆, ◆7◆, ◆9◆, ◆12◆, ◆14◆, ◆15◆, ◆16◆, and ◆19◆ (pages 31–36).

Aerobic Dance

 Start with arms out to sides, elbows at shoulder height and bent at 90-degree angles. Step sideways with right leg, bring arms together in front of you. Left leg steps next to right, arms go back to start position. Step sideways again with right, arms come together. Left foot steps next to right, arms go out to start position. Repeat to the left.

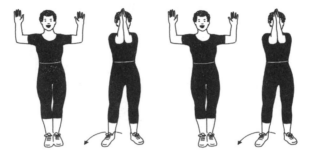

 Stepping out to side, tap foot to floor twice. As you tap, punch up twice with both arms on same side. Repeat to opposite side. Repeat sequence again, this time punching down.

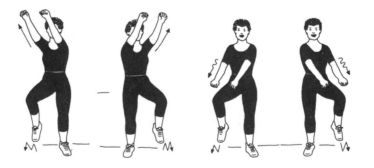

Start with hands on shoulders. Step sideways with left leg, extend palms toward ceiling. Right leg steps next to left, arms go back to start position. Step sideways again with left, extend arms up. Right leg steps next to left, back to start position. Repeat to the right.

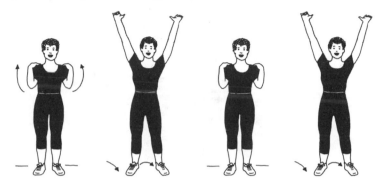

4 Start with arms at sides. Step sideways with right leg, forearms extend backward. Left leg crosses behind right, arms come up at sides, elbows bent. Step sideways with right, forearms extend back. Bring left leg next to right, arms come up. Repeat to the left.

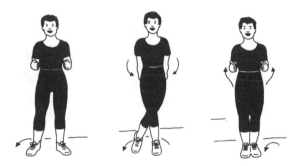

Stand in modified lunge position, right leg back, left leg bent in front. Right arm is extended back, left arm is bent and in front. Bring right leg in toward chest, bend right arm in toward chest and extend left arm back. Left leg is stationary.

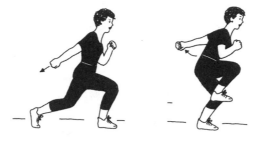

 Start with arms bent at shoulder height. Step sideways with left leg, bring elbows back. Right leg crosses behind left, arms at start position. Step sideways with left, elbows go back. Bring right leg next to left, arms at start position. Repeat to the right.

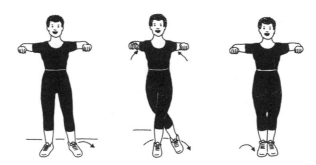

Same as 5, except start with left leg back, right leg forward.

8 Place right leg in front of left, hands on hips. Lean forward with all weight on front leg, and lift back leg. Put back leg on floor and shift body weight to back leg, lifting front.

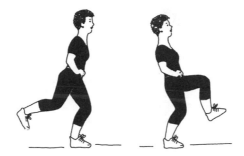

 9 Stand with arms overhead. Lift one knee, bringing arms down on either side of lifted knee. Keep back straight throughout movement. Lift other knee.

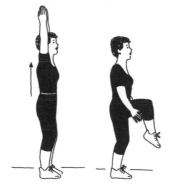

 10 Place left leg in front of right. Lean forward with all weight on front leg, and lift back leg until knee is bent, extending arms to back. Put back leg on floor and shift body weight to back leg, lifting front knee and curling arms up.

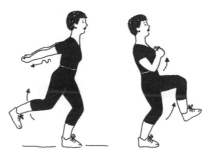

Start with arms bent and elbow at waist, hands facing forward. Kick back with bent knee, alternating legs. Each time you kick back, push arms out from chest.

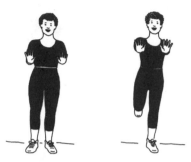

Step Aerobics

(See Aerobic Fitness Chapter [page 81] for more information about selecting a step height and general step aerobic tips.)

 Stand facing step, hands on hips. Right foot steps up. Left foot steps up with lifted knee extended over step. Left foot taps floor, lifts again and down. Right foot steps down. Left foot steps up and right foot steps up with lifted knee.

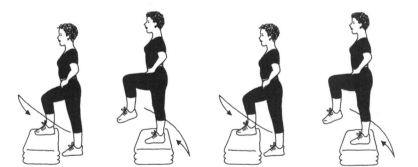

Stand facing step, hands on hips. Right foot steps up. Left foot steps up and kicks straight ahead. Left foot steps down. Right foot steps down. Left foot steps up. Right foot steps up and kicks straight ahead.

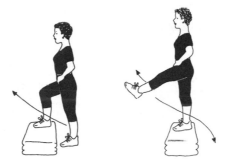

14 Same as above, except with 2 consecutive straight leg kicks.

15 Stand facing step, hands on hips. Right foot steps up on a diagonal. Left foot steps up and lifts while right hand reaches for ankle. Left foot steps down. Right foot steps down. Left foot steps up. Right foot steps up and lifts while left hand reaches for ankle.

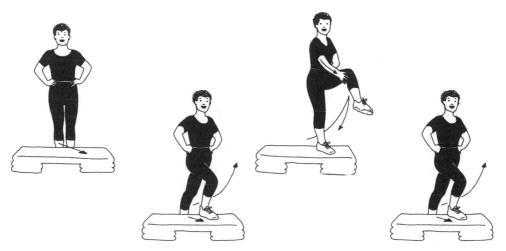

Hands on hips. Right foot steps up. Left leg extends back and up, without touching step, and returns to floor. Right foot steps down. Left foot steps up. Right leg extends up and back.

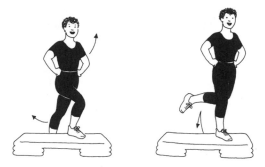

 Start with elbows bent, hands facing out at shoulder. Right foot steps up, with arms in start position. As left leg extends back and up, arms push out from chest. Left leg returns to floor, arms come in to start position. Right leg steps down, arms push out from chest. Repeat; left foot steps up with arms in at start position.

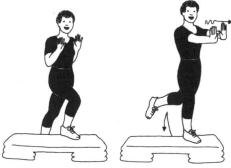

 Same as 17. Begin with arms extended at sides, bent at elbows at 90 degrees in front of body. Lift arms as left leg extends back and up.

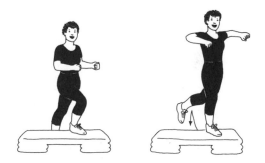

19 Same as 17. Begin with arms extended out at sides. Curl fists in toward shoulder as left leg extends back and up.

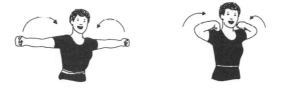

20 Place right leg on step and bend knee slightly. Left foot remains on floor. Place hands on hips. Lean forward until body weight is on right leg. Lift left leg off floor. Shift body weight to left leg and lift right foot off step. Continue with right leg on step for 20 repetitions. With practice, you'll achieve a rocking horse motion.

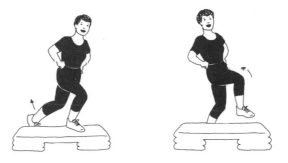

21 Same as 20, except place left leg on step and bend knee slightly.

22 Same as 20. As you place right foot on step and release weight from left leg, swing arms from sides to front of body and cross wrists out in front of you.

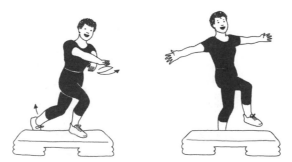

23 Bend elbows at waist. As left leg steps up and you shift weight, bring fists up toward shoulders. As weight transfers to back leg, bring arms back and down at sides.

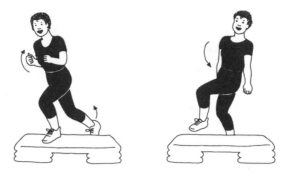

The Cardiovascular Cool-down

After a workout where you've been moving continuously, slow down the pace before your body comes to a complete stop. Spend a few minutes doing a few of the basic steps you did at the beginning of this workout at a slower pace and lighter intensity.

Toning and Strengthening

Aim for doing 15–20 reps comfortably. When you reach this point, consider adding another set or two of 15–20 reps.

Arms

 24 Sit on floor with back to step. Place hands on step, fingers pointing toward body. Keep heels on floor, and as you straighten arms, lift rest of body off floor. Slowly lower to start position.

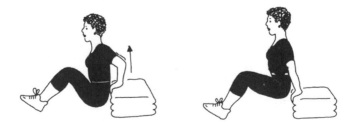

25 Face step. Bend knees and place hands on step. Keeping back straight, lower upper body toward step. (You may want to place a towel under your knees for comfort.)

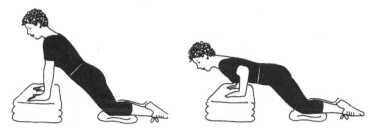

Abdominals

26 Lie on back with knees bent, heels resting on step. Cross arms over chest. Keep chin tucked to chest throughout move. Slowly roll up, lifting head, neck, and upper shoulders off floor. Hold for 10 seconds. Lower to starting position.

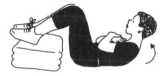

27 Lie on back on step, holding onto step at your head for support. Lift bent knees into air. (To add resistance, lower step at end where you place buttocks.)

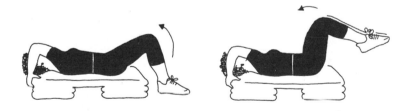

Lower back

28 Lie on stomach on step, arms and legs extended. Lift opposite arm and leg off floor. Hold for 10 seconds. Lower. Repeat with opposite arm and leg.

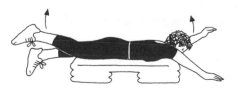

Final Cool-down

Include these stretches from Chapter 4: ◆6◆ , ◆8◆ , ◆10◆ , ◆13◆ , ◆14◆ , ◆15◆ , ◆16◆ , and ◆20◆ (pages 31–36).

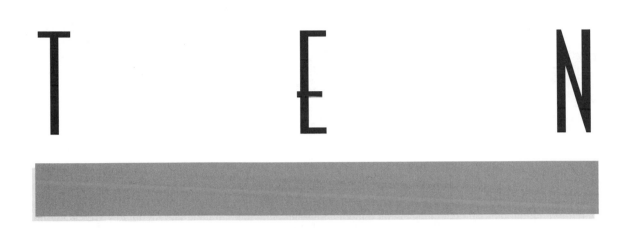

T E N

An Introduction to Other Fitness Activities

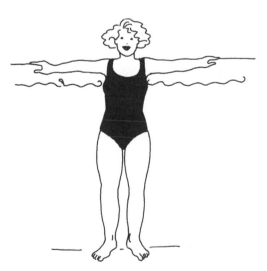

Once you begin working out and experiencing the benefits of exercise, you'll discover a world of fitness activities and sports to enjoy. Whether you're trying out a new sport, joining a health club, or purchasing home exercise equipment, you'll have the confidence and basic know-how to expand your fitness horizon. You'll also be able to take an activity you enjoy, such as cycling or swimming, and turn it into a real workout. Feeling able to take on new fitness challenges will enable you to take a break from your regular routine or try out new activities while on vacation.

Walking

As you learned in Chapter 1, you can obtain significant health benefits from exercise without exhaustive or time-consuming sessions of exercise. All you need is 30 minutes or more of moderate-intensity physical activity at least 4 days a week. While there are many ways to reach this goal, you can do it simply by walking. In fact, you can reach this goal if you walk 2 miles in 30 minutes, 4 days each week.

While this goal is easily stated, it's not easy to achieve if you haven't been active for a while. To cover 2 miles in 30 minutes requires you to walk 4 miles per hour, or 15 minutes per mile. While that's a brisk pace, it's well within your reach if you follow a personalized training program such as the one below. By following the steps outlined below, you'll be able to personalize your own walking program and comfortably reach this important health goal in a relatively short period of time.

Let your body's response determine the pace and duration of your walk.

◆ First, map out a 2-mile route (start to finish). While it's unlikely you'll be able to cover this distance right now, you'll at least have an idea of how much ground you eventually want to cover. Make sure the route is along a level surface (no significant hills or inclines). You don't need to make it more difficult if you're just getting started.

◆ Spend a few minutes doing some of the warm-up and stretching exercises pictured in Chapter Four, starting on page 27 (focus on stretching your leg muscles). This warm-up will help to loosen tight muscles and joints, decreasing your chances of aches, pains, or cramps during or after your session.

- Always start out slowly! Even if you're in good shape, spend the first few minutes of your walk at a slower pace. This gives your cardiovascular system a chance to get "warmed up" for the more challenging work that follows.

- Pick up the pace, walking at the speed you find most comfortable. Strive to cover as much of the 2-mile distance as you *comfortably* can (be sure to consider the return leg of your walk). Don't be concerned if your pace is slower than other individuals you may see while out walking. What is important is that you feel comfortable throughout your walk!

- Don't complete your walk without slowing down first! Before coming to a complete stop, slow your pace. This "cool-down" period gives your body a chance to readjust to a resting level gradually.

- Repeat some of the stretching exercises you did while warming up to complete your workout.

Over the next few weeks, follow the guidelines outlined below, based on the results of your first walk.

You Were Able to Cover the Full 2 Miles; However, It Took More Than 30 Minutes

In future workouts, strive to walk faster even if you can sustain it for only a minute or two before returning to your regular pace. A good strategy is to alternate ever-increasing periods of faster walking with decreasing periods of regular walking. Soon your regular pace will be faster!

You Were Unable to Cover the Full 2-Mile Distance

Maintaining your regular pace, strive to cover more ground during each workout. Over time (it may take a few weeks), strive to cover the full 2 miles without trying to walk any faster. When you're able to go for the full 2 miles, then try to pick up the pace. Follow the guidelines outlined above to cover the full 2 miles in 30 minutes.

Ready for Jogging: How to Incorporate Jogging into Your Walk

Jogging not only burns a lot of calories in a relatively short period of time, but it can also boost your level of cardiovascular fitness. When are you ready for jogging? There are no set rules, but if you're interested in jogging and can comfortably walk continuously for 45 to 60 minutes, then you're ready to add some jogging to your sessions of walking. To get started:

◆ Complete your regular warm-up and flexibility exercises, then set out on your usual walk.

◆ When you reach a street crossing, jog lightly across the street. When you reach the opposite sidewalk, resume walking. (If you walk on a path or around a track, use a distance similar to streets and blocks as markers for walking and jogging.)

◆ Continue jogging across streets and walking on sidewalks.

◆ Finish up the session with walking, and continue your cool-down by repeating the stretching exercises you did while warming up.

◆ Over the next few weeks as your capacity for jogging improves (that is, you're breathing easier), start jogging before reaching the street crossing, and continue past the start of the sidewalk on the opposite side of the street. As the weeks pass, add more steps of jogging and reduce the time you spend walking. Soon you'll be able to jog continuously from start to finish. (Note: when you get to this point, it's time to switch from good walking shoes to a pair of good running shoes.)

Cycling

How to Turn a Bike Ride into a Workout

◆ Before setting out, make sure your bike is in working order. Always wear a helmet to protect your head. (Some states now require all cyclists to wear helmets.)

◆ Plan a route along level ground. Going up too many hills will quickly tire you out. Going down too many hills doesn't give you a chance to pedal—gravity does the work for you.

◆ Before getting on the bike, spend a few minutes doing some of the warm-up and stretching exercises pictured in Chapter Four, starting on page 27, focusing on stretching your leg muscles.

◆ Start off slowly. Find a comfortable pedaling speed. Don't be concerned with how fast you go; it's how long you keep going that's important.

◆ If you're feeling a little fatigued

Pedal a little less and coast a little more.

Pedal a little slower.

Change gears to make pedaling easier.

◆ Continue cycling as long as you comfortably can (and be sure to consider the return part of your ride).

◆ Before ending your workout, it's important to spend the last few minutes "cooling down." Pedal a little slower or change gears to make pedaling easier, but either way, keep pedaling. Stopping a session of cycling abruptly can make you feel dizzy or light-headed.

◆ Repeat some of the stretching exercises you did while warming up to complete your workout.

How to Keep Cycling Challenging

◆ Gradually increase the amount of time you spend cycling by doing one of the following:

Increasing the length of your typical workout

Increasing the number of workouts per week

Increasing both the frequency and length of your cycling workouts

◆ As you approach the upper limit of time you can devote to cycling, focus your attention on working progressively harder in future workouts. Use one or more of the following strategies:

Add some reasonable hills to your typical route.

Change gears to make pedaling more difficult.

Pedal more, coast less.

Pedal a little faster.

◆ Because you'll be working harder in each workout, you may get tired sooner and your typical workout may be shorter. As the weeks progress, attempt to increase the duration of each workout to the limit you've set aside for cycling.

Swimming

How to Make Swimming a Workout

◆ As with any exercise session, start off by warming up. Before getting into the pool, or while standing in the shallow water, spend a few minutes doing some of the warm-up and stretching exercises pictured in Chapter Four, starting on page 27, focusing on your arms and legs.

◆ Start off slowly. Swim your favorite stroke for the first lap. Listen to your body: Can you *comfortably* swim the return lap without taking a short rest? If you feel you need a rest, consider the following options until you feel ready for the next lap:

Get out of the pool, walk to the other end, and begin swimming again.

If you're in the deep end, hold on to the side of the pool and try some flutter or scissors kicks.

If you're in the shallow end, walk around in the shallow water.

◆ When you're ready for your next lap, turn around and begin swimming. If you would like to ease up a bit, swim this lap with a less vigorous stroke—the elementary back stroke, side stroke, and breast-stroke contain a "glide" or rest phase, making them a little less taxing.

◆ Swim as many laps as you comfortably can. Remember, your laps need not be continuous. Don't hesitate to rest when you feel the need for a break. Use some of the strategies noted above to keep active while you take a break from swimming.

◆ Before getting out of the pool, spend the last few minutes engaged in gradually less strenuous activities. You can "cool down" by

Slowing down the pace of your swimming

Swimming less vigorous strokes

Walking around in the shallow water

Holding onto the side of the pool and kicking your legs

◆ Repeat some of the stretching exercises you did while warming up to complete your workout.

How to Keep Your Swimming Challenging

◆ Over the next few weeks, gradually spend more time in the pool by:

Increasing the duration of your typical workout

Increasing the number of workouts per week

Increasing both the frequency and length of your swimming workouts

◆ As you approach the upper limit of time you can devote to swimming, strive to:

String together an ever-increasing number of laps before you have to rest

Gradually reduce the number of strokes you swim that contain a "glide" phase—swim more and more vigorous strokes

◆ Because you'll be working harder in each workout, you may fatigue sooner and your typical workout will be shortened. As the weeks progress, attempt to increase the duration of each workout toward the limit you've set aside for swimming.

Tips on Choosing Home Exercise Equipment

Thinking about buying exercise equipment to be used at home? See the chart on pages 120–121. There are so many choices—stationary bicycles, treadmills, rowing machines, mini-gyms. How do you know what's best for you? Before considering the attributes of each kind of equipment, and what to look for when making a purchase, consider these questions:

What Are Your Exercise Goals? What Purpose Do You Want the Equipment to Serve?

Keep the answer to these questions in mind as you shop for equipment. If the equipment you see is not specifically designed to help you reach your goal, it's not for you! For example, if your concern is to tone up your muscles, don't waste your time looking at treadmills—a mini-gym should be the focus of your attention.

Home Exercise Equipment Pros and Cons

	Primary Focus	*What to Look for*
Stationary Cycle	• Burn calories • Aerobic fitness • Tone thighs	• Only consider models with a mechanism allowing you to control how difficult it is to pedal. • Apply a modest amount of resistance and try to pedal. The pedaling motion should be smooth —not jerky or sticky. • The seat should be wide and well padded (comfortable). Its height must be adjustable.
Treadmill	• Burn calories • Aerobic fitness	• Easy to reach push-button controls to regulate speed and elevation. • The motor should generate at least 1.5 horsepower. • Adjustments to speed and elevation should be made with a smooth and even response. • The platform should be long and wide enough for your walking or running style.
Rowing Machine	• Burn calories • Aerobic fitness • Tone all major muscle groups	• Check the movement of the seat while seated in it. The seat should slide back and forth freely without sticking. • Rowing motion should remain smooth and fluid with the application of added resistance.
Mini-Gym	• Tone and strengthen muscles • Circuit resistance training burns significant calories	• A sturdy, stable frame is essential. • Changing from one exercise station to another should require minimal time and effort. Likewise, modifying the resistance should be easy to accomplish. • Make sure the gym offers the ability to work the muscles you want to tone.
Cross-Country Ski Simulator	• Burn calories • Aerobic fitness	• Skis that move independently—the movement of one should not force the movement of the other. • Test the action of the skis while standing in them. Their movement should be smooth and stable. • The ability to adjust the resistance to arm and leg movements

Advantages	Disadvantages	General Comments
• Because your weight is supported by the seat, cycling places little strain on the weight-bearing joints.	• Some find this activity boring. It can be made more enjoyable if done while watching TV, listening to music, or reading (consider purchasing a reading stand).	• Dual-action cycles (exercise both arms and legs) can provide a more vigorous workout and help to tone the muscles of the arms and chest.
• Allows you to walk or even jog in the privacy and comfort of your home. • Easier on your joints (better shock absorption) than running on a road or other hard and uneven surface.	• Price. Quality treadmills are expensive	• Treadmills are sophisticated pieces of equipment. If you can't afford to purchase a good one, it's best to consider another piece of home exercise equipment.
• Because you are seated, rowing, like cycling, is easy on the weight-bearing joints.	• Because proper form is so important (arm and leg movements must be coordinated), rowing requires a degree of skill.	• If you have a history of back problems, check with your physician before making a purchase.
• Effectively tones all major muscle groups. • Generally safer and easier than working with free weights.	• In an effort to offer all exercises in one machine, • Some of the exercises may be a bit unconventional. • Some models require significant floor space. • Price. Mini-gyms can be expensive.	• If your primary goal is to improve muscle tone and strength, a mini-gym is your best bet.
• Provides a superior aerobic workout yet the smooth gliding motion is easy on your joints.	• Requires a higher level of skill (coordination of arm and leg movements) than other pieces of home exercise equipment.	• Because this activity is so demanding, it should not be considered by individuals not already exercising on a regular basis.

To Date, Have You Been Successful Making Time in Your Schedule to Exercise?

If the answer is yes, there is a good chance you'll also be successful finding time to use home exercise equipment. If, on the other hand, the answer is no, be sure the home exercise equipment increases the likelihood you'll exercise more frequently. That is, it should help overcome an obstacle that prevents you from exercising on a regular basis.

General Prepurchasing Tips

◆ Take a test run, row, or pedal. Make sure the machine fits your body size and shape.

◆ High-tech gadgetry (computer-simulated rides, heart rate monitors, or caloric expenditure displays) generally add to the cost while not always providing significant value.

◆ Ask if the dealer or manufacturer offers a warranty. The answer should provide insight regarding durability and maintenance.

◆ Stores generally have floor models. Check to see how they have stood up to use.

Choosing an Exercise Facility

While it isn't necessary to join an exercise facility to get fit or to control your weight, many people find that it's easier for them to achieve their exercise goals with the proper equipment, classes, and staff available at these facilities.

Review your personal exercise goals. Do exercise facilities provide services that will help you to meet these goals? If the answer is "yes" and you're interested in joining one, keep these factors in mind as you shop for an exercise facility:

Service Offerings

As you shop for an exercise facility, your most immediate concern must be to make sure the services and/or equipment available will help you to meet your exercise goals. In addition, you'll want to consider the availability of activities and equipment you may want to use in the future—as your fitness level increases.

Convenience

The closer a facility is to home or to work, the better. It's always easy to find an excuse not to exercise if getting to the facility takes you out of your way or off the "beaten path." Steer clear of exercise facilities that require a long, out-of-the-way drive or classes/hours that don't easily fit your schedule.

Staff Qualifications

Before joining, ask about the staff's educational background and/or certifications. CPR certification is a must. Educational backgrounds in physical education or certification from a nationally recognized exercise organization is expected. You should also get a feel for the number of staff members on duty at a given time. Does this number seem adequate?

Facilities and Equipment

Consider whether the facility has the types of equipment and/or services you need to reach your exercise goals. If it does, are they available in numbers sufficient to prevent overcrowding? Look for signs that a facility is underequipped, overcrowded, or mismanaged. Ask for a tour of the activity areas as well as the locker room (ideally at the time you plan to use the club). Determine whether the facility and its equipment are well maintained and clean and try to observe whether all advertised equipment is present.

Safety

When you visit an exercise facility, you should have the feeling that member safety is the number-one concern of its management and staff. A pre-activity screening questionnaire and/or medical history form should be completed before you're allowed to participate in any activity. A provision for a personal demonstration of the equipment is important. Well-maintained exercise equipment, adequate floor space, and first aid equipment are other visible signs of this commitment to member safety.

General Business

See and experience as much as you can before committing yourself to any type of membership or contract. Is a trial membership or guest pass available? If not, ask whether a short-term membership is available. Be sure you understand precisely what your membership fee entitles you to. Are there extra fees for use of specific services or facilities (for example, the swimming pool, tennis courts, lessons, fitness testing services)? Request a copy of the rules and regulations regarding use of the facilities. Be sure not to sign a contract until all your questions are answered to your satisfaction.

Finding the Best Aerobic Dance Class

If you prefer to work out with a group or find the motivation of an instructor keeps you going, consider taking an aerobic dance class. But before signing up, check the following:

◆ Does it look like fun? Talk to the instructor and observe a class before signing up. Watch out for "killer aerobics" that can cause injuries; gentler, moderate classes are usually best.

◆ Does the instructor have the educational background and/or certification from a recognized professional organization to lead the class? It's a fair question to ask the instructor or the management of the facility.

◆ Is the class size manageable? Not only is overcrowding unsafe, but you may not receive the attention and instruction you deserve. Don't get lost in the crowd!

◆ Does the dance floor have some give? Concrete or tile is too hard, a wooden floor over a compressible base is best. Dancing on too hard a floor puts undue stress on your joints and bones.

In addition, the instructor should:

◆ Encourage you to "do what you comfortably can" and not force you to follow the crowd

◆ Take the time to demonstrate new steps adequately

◆ Demonstrate modifications to steps that allow you to regulate the intensity of the routine, making it more or less strenuous to suit your needs

Exercise in the Water for Nonswimmers

Even if you can't swim, just walking or exercising in the water can provide significant benefits. For those with weak legs or painful ankle, knee, or hip joints, exercising in the water is much more comfortable than exercising on land. The buoyancy provided by the water helps to reduce the weight your joints support and carry. Check with your local Y or swimming pool for the availability of nonswimmer exercise classes. Use some of the exercises pictured on pages 125–127 and put together your own mini workout.

Use these exercises to burn calories and improve aerobic fitness:

1 Standing in waist-to-chest-deep water, simulate overhand crawl stroke by reaching out with left hand, getting a "grip" on the water, pressing downward and pulling, bringing left hand through to thigh. Reach out with right hand and repeat.

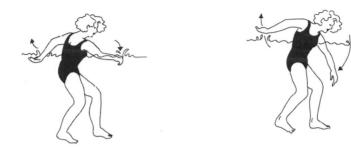

2 With fingers laced behind neck, walk forward, bringing up alternate legs and twisting body to touch knees with opposite elbow. Repeat.

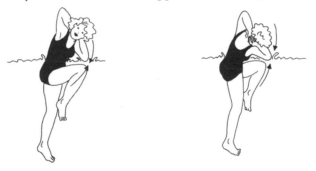

3 Standing in chest-deep water, bounce on left foot, at same time pushing down vigorously with both hands, causing upper body to rise. Repeat with other leg.

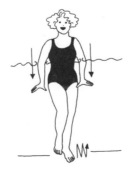

Standing in waist-deep water, bounce in place with high knee action. Keep right arm outstretched far forward when left knee is high. Stretch left arm and hand rearward. Repeat on other side. When bringing right arm back, pull down and through with arm simulating crawl stroke.

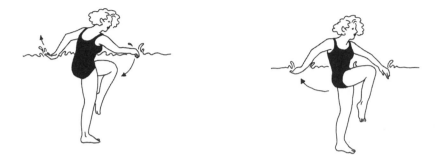

 Standing with arms bent in running position, jog in place.

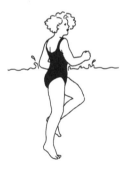

Use these exercises to tone and strength abdominal muscles:

Lying back and holding onto pool gutter with knees drawn up to chest, twist slowly to left, recover, twist slowly to right, recover. Repeat on other side.

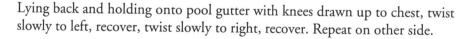
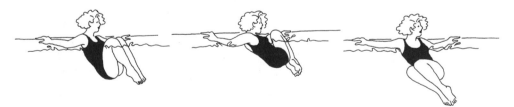

7 Lying back and holding onto pool gutter with legs extended, swing legs far apart, then bring legs together, crossing left leg over right. Repeat, crossing right over left.

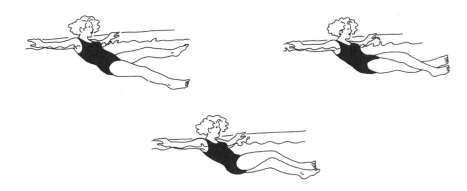

8 Standing, holding onto pool gutter with hands, back to wall, lift left knee and cross it over other leg, twisting to right, recover. Repeat with other leg.

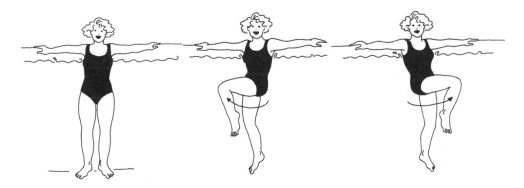

Recreational Activities and Sports

Recreational activities and sports provide fun and companionship and yield fitness benefits—whether it's aerobic fitness, muscle conditioning, or flexibility. Once you develop the skills you need on the tennis court, or on cross-country skis, for example, you could be on your way to acquiring an enjoyable lifelong activity. Following are six popular sports, their benefits, and their pros and cons.

Tennis

Benefits

Skilled players expend significant calories. Playing singles requires more running, and generally provides a more vigorous workout. Beginners can also get a workout from skill-building drills (for example, hitting with an instructor or hitting off a practice wall).

Advantages

A social sport. Most communities have public courts.

Disadvantages

Playing out of season requires use of an indoor court, which often requires a fee. Hard to control exercise intensity.

Racquetball

Benefits

Skilled players burn lots of calories. As in squash, racquetball requires that you hit a small ball inside a boxlike four-walled court. Although the racquet is shorter than either tennis or squash the sport requires similar skills and yields comparable benefits.

Advantages

Easier to learn than tennis.

Disadvantages

It will cost you a few dollars to play. Some health clubs have racquetball courts; other court-only clubs require a membership fee or pay-as-you-play cost. Hard to control exercise intensity.

Golf

Benefits

Main health benefit is walking the course, not swinging the club.

Advantages

A social sport played in pleasant outdoor surroundings.

Disadvantages

Because of the popularity of the sport, many courses require you to use a golf cart to speed up play and accommodate those waiting their turn. Requires a significant level of skill before you're ready to get out on the course.

Hiking

Benefits

Health benefit is similar to walking, but because hiking is done on trails, mountains, or other rough terrain, it does more to strengthen leg muscles and burns more calories than walking. Also, carrying a backpack adds to the demands of this activity.

Advantages

An inexpensive and pleasant outdoor activity. The only special equipment required is a well-fitted hiking shoe.

Disadvantages

Be aware of safety. Don't hike alone, and always carry drinking water and a first aid kit. Trail safety depends on where you are and on weather, climate, and season.

Skating

Benefits

In-line skating (often known as rollerblading) or ice skating can give you an aerobic workout if your skating is continuous. Skating also strengthens legs and buttocks.

Advantages

The same basic gliding movement is required for both in-line and ice skating, so if you like in-line skating, you may find ice skating a pleasant winter activity. Today's in-line skates are made of hard plastic and give the ankle more support than leather upper ice skates.

Disadvantages

Before you invest in a pair of skates, rent them first to see if you like the sport. Make sure you consider the cost of safety equipment—helmet and pads—before buying skates.

Cross-Country Skiing

Benefits

Skilled skiers burn significant calories, improve aerobic fitness, and build muscles in the upper and lower body.

Advantages

A family or group activity. On cross-country trails you can get off the main roads and explore beautiful countryside.

Disadvantages

Limited access to good conditions is based on the season and where you live. Requires a greater level of skill than most traditional aerobic activities.

E L E V E N

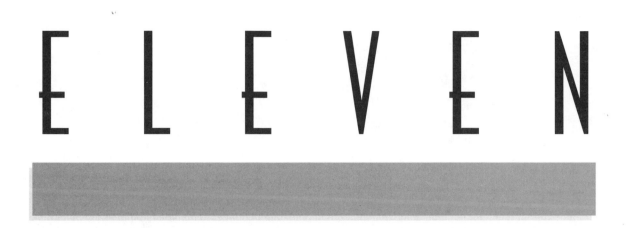

Personal Fitness Planner

Use the planners here to record your weekly activity. Assess your progress with the chart on page 134.

Current Fitness Goal:

Check one box:

❑ to lose or control your weight   ❑ to improve flexibility

❑ to improve muscular strength   ❑ multiple fitness goals
and tone

❑ to improve cardiovascular fitness

Goal for this week is: _____

To increase my chances of reaching this goal, I'll take these steps:

1.

2.

3.

Fill in the appropriate number of minutes you spent this week on workouts or other activities:

Workout/Activity	Mon	Tues	Wed	Thurs	Fri	Sat	Sun
Calorie-Burning*							
Toning and Strengthening*							
Flexibility and Stress Reduction*							
Aerobic*							
Overall Workout*							
Walking							
Walking-jogging							
Cycling							
Swimming							
Exercise in water							
Tennis							
Racquetball							
Hiking							
Skating							
Cross-country skiing							
Other activity or sport							

*Workouts in *Weight Watchers Complete Exercise Book*

Current Fitness Goal:

Check one box:

❏ to lose or control your weight   ❏ to improve flexibility

❏ to improve muscular strength   ❏ multiple fitness goals
and tone

❏ to improve cardiovascular fitness

Goal for this week is: _____

To increase my chances of reaching this goal, I'll take these steps:

1.

2.

3.

Fill in the appropriate number of minutes you spent this week on workouts or other activities:

Workout/Activity	Mon	Tues	Wed	Thurs	Fri	Sat	Sun
Calorie-Burning*	____	____	____	____	____	____	____
Toning and Strengthening*	____	____	____	____	____	____	____
Flexibility and Stress Reduction*	____	____	____	____	____	____	____
Aerobic*	____	____	____	____	____	____	____
Overall Workout*	____	____	____	____	____	____	____
Walking	____	____	____	____	____	____	____
Walking-jogging	____	____	____	____	____	____	____
Cycling	____	____	____	____	____	____	____
Swimming	____	____	____	____	____	____	____
Exercise in water	____	____	____	____	____	____	____
Tennis	____	____	____	____	____	____	____
Racquetball	____	____	____	____	____	____	____
Hiking	____	____	____	____	____	____	____
Skating	____	____	____	____	____	____	____
Cross-country skiing	____	____	____	____	____	____	____
Other activity or sport	____	____	____	____	____	____	____

*Workouts in *Weight Watchers Complete Exercise Book*

Forward with Fitness

To get perspective on how your fitness is improving, compare your current activity level to before you began your regular exercise program. (Don't compare yourself to anyone but yourself!) Examine what you did during a typical day in the past and compare it with your current level of activity. Use the list below to focus your attention on specific habits. (Not all the items listed below will apply to your specific situation.)

Determine whether, during a typical week, you spend more, less, or the same amount of time doing the activities listed below. Mark each item as follows:

+   (more)

—   (less)

NC   (no change)

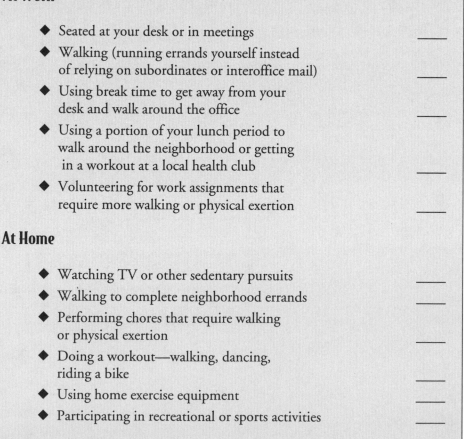

At Work

◆ Seated at your desk or in meetings _____

◆ Walking (running errands yourself instead of relying on subordinates or interoffice mail) _____

◆ Using break time to get away from your desk and walk around the office _____

◆ Using a portion of your lunch period to walk around the neighborhood or getting in a workout at a local health club _____

◆ Volunteering for work assignments that require more walking or physical exertion _____

At Home

◆ Watching TV or other sedentary pursuits _____

◆ Walking to complete neighborhood errands _____

◆ Performing chores that require walking or physical exertion _____

◆ Doing a workout—walking, dancing, riding a bike _____

◆ Using home exercise equipment _____

◆ Participating in recreational or sports activities _____

When assessing your progress, don't expect to see positive changes everywhere, just where it makes sense for you. It's wise to make small, modest changes that you can build into your lifestyle rather than drastic changes that are harder to stick with. If you've become active in just one area of your life, you're on your way to a healthier you!

INDEX